Advances in Experimental Medicine and Biology

Volume 1216

Advances in Experimental Medicine and Biology presents multidisciplinary and dynamic findings in the broad fields of experimental medicine and biology. The wide variety in topics it presents offers readers multiple perspectives on a variety of disciplines including neuroscience, microbiology, immunology, biochemistry, biomedical engineering and cancer research.

Advances in Experimental Medicine and Biology has been publishing exceptional works in the field for over 30 years and is indexed in SCOPUS; Medline (PubMed); Journal Citation Reports/Science Edition; Science Citation Index Expanded (SciSearch) (Web of Science); EMBASE; BIOSIS; Reaxys; EMBiology; Chemical Abstracts Service (CAS); Pathway Studio. The series also provides scientists with up to date information on emerging topics and techniques.

2018 Impact Factor: 2.126.

More information about this series at http://www.springer.com/series/5584

Nicola Veronese
Editor

Frailty and Cardiovascular Diseases

Research into an Elderly Population

Springer

Editor
Nicola Veronese
National Research Council
Neuroscience Institute, Aging Branch
Padova, Italy

ISSN 0065-2598 ISSN 2214-8019 (electronic)
Advances in Experimental Medicine and Biology
ISBN 978-3-030-33329-4 ISBN 978-3-030-33330-0 (eBook)
https://doi.org/10.1007/978-3-030-33330-0

This Springer imprint is published by the registered company Springer Nature Switzerland AG
The registered company address is: Gewerbestrasse 11, 6330 Cham, Switzerland

Preface

Frailty and cardiovascular diseases (CVD) are two common conditions in the elderly, highly affecting clinical outcomes in older people. Epidemiological studies suggest that CVD are among the most relevant contributors in the development of frailty. At the same time, increasing research is showing that frailty can be considered as a potential CVD risk factor, independently from other CVD risk factors. The association between CVD and frailty is probably due to the shared etiological factors, including low-grade inflammation, cellular senescence, and endocrine dysregulation. The early detection of frailty is therefore important in the management of patients with CVD or in people who are at high risk of having CVD, such as frail patients. In this regard, the use of a comprehensive geriatric assessment (CGA) seems to be essential for better taking care of older people with CVD or in those at high risk for developing CVD.

In this book, we will offer to the reader an overview of the current evidence regarding the epidemiology of frailty and CVD and their co-existence in terms of epidemiological research. Moreover, some chapters will be dedicated to exploring the underlying pathophysiology, with a special interest on inflammation and oxidative stress. Finally, the clinical importance of frailty in CVD and vice versa will be discussed. A last part will be dedicated to the treatment of frailty and CVD and the newer topics of interest in this field.

Therefore, this book will offer an up-to-date review on the potential relationship between frailty and CVD, which may represent a novel topic in geriatric medicine. Accordingly, the book will be relevant to a wide range of clinicians. The authorship will include many of the best known and widely published experts in their respective fields.

Nicola Veronese
National Research Council
Neuroscience Institute, Aging Branch
Padova, Italy

Primary Care Department, Geriatric Unit
Geriatric Unit, Azienda ULSS 3 (Unità Locale Socio Sanitaria)
Dolo-Mirano District, Venice, Italy

Contents

1 Frailty: What Is It?

Marco Proietti and Matteo Cesari

Abstract

Over the past decades, a progressive and exponential aging of the population has been observed. In particular, an absolute e relative increase of old and very old persons is also projected for the next 30 years. This demographic phenomenon is substantially responsible for the growing prevalence of frailty in our societies. Frailty is a clinical condition characterized by an excessive vulnerability of the individual to endogenous and exogenous stressors. This status generates a high risk of developing negative health-related events. Shifting to a construct as frailty to biologically define the perimeter of action for geriatric medicine will probably concur at modernizing the old way of practicing medicine. In this chapter the concept of frailty, its impact on the evolving healthcare systems, the controversies associated with its assessment and, ultimately, the role it plays in the management of older persons are discussed.

Keywords

Elderly · Frailty · Ageing · Geriatric assessment

1.1 Introduction

Over the past decades, a progressive aging of the population has been observed worldwide. It is noteworthy that the number of old and very old individuals has substantially increased both in absolute and relative terms. Furthermore, demographic projections show that the growth of older age groups is expected to continue for the next 30 years (United Nations 2015).

The aging of our societies contributes at critically challenging the sustainability of the healthcare systems. In fact, older persons are characterized by high clinical complexity (with consequent polypharmacy), disabling conditions, and social issues (National Institute for Health and Care Excellence 2017; Masnoon et al. 2017; Payne 2016). All these factors make the older population quite different from the standards upon which the healthcare systems were originally designed (Tinetti and Fried 2004). In particular, the fragmentation of care services and the rigid disease-centered approach determine a relevant gap between the person's priorities/needs and the provided responses.

M. Proietti (✉) · M. Cesari
Department of Clinical Sciences and Community Health, University of Milan, Milan, Italy
e-mail: marco.proietti@unimi.it

M. Proietti · M. Cesari
Geriatric Unit, Fondazione IRCCS Ca' Granda Ospedale Maggiore Policlinico, Milan, Italy

N. Veronese (ed.), *Frailty and Cardiovascular Diseases*, Advances in Experimental Medicine and Biology 1216, https://doi.org/10.1007/978-3-030-33330-0_1

In order to adapt the traditional clinical and research approach to the new (older) older population referring to our services, several theoretical constructs have been proposed in the geriatric literature. Special attention in this context has to be reserved to frailty (Cesari et al. 2017a).

Despite the existence of a largely agreed definition of frailty (i.e., a medical condition characterized by the reduction of homeostatic reserves, exposing the individual to higher vulnerability to stressors and risk of negative health-related outcomes (Morley et al. 2013)), its definition remains controversial (WHO 2015). It is paradigmatic a systematic review of the literature published in 2016 by Buta and colleagues, which listed more than 60 validated instruments for measuring frailty (Buta et al. 2016).

In this chapter, the condition of frailty is presented in its theoretical and operational features. Moreover, its clinical and research relevance as well as the controversies associated with its assessment are discussed.

1.2 The Concept of Frailty

In a consensus statement published in 2013, six major international scientific societies (International Association of Gerontology and Geriatrics; Society on Sarcopenia, Cachexia, and Wasting Diseases; International Academy of Nutrition and Aging; European Geriatric Medicine Society; American Medical Directors Association; American Federation for Aging Research) endorsed the definition of frailty as "a medical syndrome with multiple causes and contributors that is characterized by diminished strength, endurance, and reduced physiologic function that increases an individual's vulnerability for developing increased dependency and/or death" (Morley et al. 2013). This definition stands on specific theoretical pillars. In particular, it is established that frailty is different from disability, sarcopenia, and/or multimorbidity. In other words, although a frail subject can be disabled, may present sarcopenia, and/or affected by multiple diseases, none of these three conditions can comprehensively capture the concept of frailty; they may just represent specific aspects of such complex age-related condition (Morley et al. 2013). It was also explained that frailty may find its causal roots in the physical or cognitive domains of the individual (Morley et al. 2013). Frailty was also described as a dynamic entity able to improve or worsen over time.

A growing body of the literature has recently focused on multimorbidity as a parallel concept to frailty. Both are, in fact, designed to capture the clinical complexity of the aging person. Multimorbidity is defined as the coexistence of two or more chronic diseases, not related each other, in the same individual (National Institute for Health and Care Excellence 2017; Mannucci and Nobili 2014). Multimorbidity has attracted a lot of interest in the scientific community, and several societies have provided specific guidance on its management (National Institute for Health and Care Excellence 2017; Muth et al. 2019). Multimorbidity is associated with increased risk for adverse health-related outcomes (Castro et al. 2017; Fraccaro et al. 2016; Barnett et al. 2012). By counting the number of diseases, it is assumed that a more comprehensive assessment and holistic approach to the individual will be possible. Multimorbidity moves from the single-disease approach to a vision characterized by the simultaneous existence of multiple nosological conditions (to be organized and treated) (Cesari et al. 2016a, 2017b).

Frailty and multimorbidity are closely related (Vetrano et al. 2018) and often been alternatively used (as wrongly considered synonymous). Instead, a clear difference exists between them (Cesari et al. 2017b). Whereas multimorbidity relies upon the mono-dimensional construct of disease (i.e., nosologically defined conditions), frailty potentially implies a more exhaustive and comprehensive assessment of the individual (including signs, symptoms, clinical conditions, disabilities). The geriatric background of the former is evident, especially if considering how difficult is to complete a diagnostic *iter* in older persons due to clinical, functional, cost-effectiveness, social, and ethical issues.

The concept of frailty is very close to the resilience one. Resilience is described as the human ability to adapt when a traumatic life stressor suddenly occurs (Morley et al. 2013). On a purely theoretical basis, the same stressor will generate heterogeneous consequences in different individuals. Therefore, a resilient person will be able to completely restore his/her health status after a negative stressor in a relatively short time, whereas a poorly resilient individual will struggle to restore the *quo ante* condition and will also take more time to recover.

Interestingly, the World Health Organization (WHO) published in 2015 the 'World Report on Ageing and Health'. In this document, the novel concept of intrinsic capacity was theoretically framed and presented (WHO 2015). Intrinsic capacity is here defined as the composite of all the physical and mental capacities of an individual. By interacting with the environment, intrinsic capacity determines the functional ability of the individual, that is the health-related attributes that enable people to be and to do what they have reason to value (WHO 2015). Intrinsic capacity and functional capacity tend to diverge with advancing age. The environment becomes more and more burdening on the capacity of the person to function at his/her best. The document thus insists on the importance of reducing the environmental barriers and/or increasing the intrinsic capacity by levering on the individual's reserves in order to promote the optimal functional ability. It is noteworthy that this novel framework is largely based on the background literature of frailty. In fact, although differences between frailty and intrinsic capacity are quite evident, the two concepts are both (1) designed to promote a novel and comprehensive approach to the aging individual, and (2) based on the necessary integration of care services.

1.3 The Assessment of Frailty

Several tools exist to measure frailty and the number of validated tools has steadily increased over the years (Cesari et al. 2017a). Table 1.1 presents the most commonly known tools, although the list is far to be exhaustive (Buta et al. 2016).

Among the different models of frailty, two major school of thoughts might be identified in the literature. Probably, the most commonly known is the model of the frailty phenotype proposed by Fried and colleagues (Fried et al. 2001), based on five signs/symptoms (i.e. weight loss, fatigue, weakness, slowness, reduced or absent physical activity).

Differently, Rockwood and Mitnitski proposed in 2001 the so-called "age-related accumulation of deficits" model of frailty (Mitnitski et al. 2001). It is based on the concept that aging is a continuous process characterized by the accumulation of deficits. Its operationalization gives life to the Frailty Index (FI).

The frailty phenotype and the FI are clearly different. The frailty underlying them is not the same. The frailty phenotype presents a clinical manifestation based on five predefined signs/symptoms. It is not necessary to adequately know the individual for observing this physical evidence. Differently, the FI consider frailty as a heterogeneous state captured during the aging process. It requires a comprehensive assessment of the person for computing the FI, which may consequently resemble a surrogate of biological age.

Independently of the instrument used to measure frailty, it is always important to contextualize the assessment with the subsequent actions. If the detection of frailty is not able to modify the clinician's decisional algorithm, then the assessment is useless (Cesari et al. 2017a).

1.4 Frailty and Disability

As discussed, a controversy exists around the concept of frailty. One of the major issues in this field can be found in the positioning of frailty in relation to disability (i.e., the functional limitation of the individual in the accomplishment of activities of daily living (Cesari et al. 2017b)). Although Fried and colleagues did not exclude the possibility that frailty and disability might co-exist, the condition captured by the frailty phenotype has often been considered as a sort of "pre-disability" disability (Fried et al. 2011). This is probably due to the fact that most studies

Table 1.1 Examples of validated instruments for the screening and assessment of frailty (Cesari et al. 2016a; Morley et al. 2013)

Author	Model
Fried (2001)	Frailty Phenotype
Mitnitski (2001)	Frailty index
Schuurmans (2004)	Groningen frailty index
Rockwood (2005)	Clinical frailty scale
Ensrud (2008)	Study of osteoporotic fractures index
Romero-Ortuno (2010)	SHARE frailty instrument
Gobbens (2010)	Tilburg frailty index
Morley (2012)	FRAIL
Pilotto (2012)	Multi-prognostic index
Mossello (2016)	INTER-FRAIL

have used the phenotype to capture a risk condition for incident disability. On the other hand, disabilities can be part of the frailty status captured by the deficit accumulation model.

This issue is not trivial, especially if it is taken into account the relevance that disability has for geriatric medicine. If disability is left outside of frailty, then frailty may become the key target for preventive interventions against disability. It means anticipating the geriatric practice to the community, where frail non-disabled individuals live. On the other hand, by accepting that disability is included under the frailty umbrella does not necessarily anticipate, but surely redefine the perimeter of action for geriatric medicine (having biological age as criterion to set the target).

As discussed elsewhere, the interactions of frailty, multimorbidity, and disability may give life to three main scenarios:

- Phenotype model. In this model, the three entities are considered at the same level and independent each other. They can coexist and overlap. A person can thus be at the same time multimorbid, disable, and frail (as suggested by Fried and colleagues in (Fried et al. 2011));
- Pre-disability model. Frailty and multimorbidity act as risk factors for disability. This latter represents the endpoint of interest, and a methodological choice is driving the decision of considering frailty (with/without multimorbidity) as a pre-disability condition;
- Model for adapted care. Frailty is here considered in a broader sense, that is as a condition of public health interest. Frailty is here a biological condition of accentuated vulnerability, where multimorbidity and disability may serve as contributors. In other words, multimorbidity and disability are "contained" within the concept of frailty, as suggested by the FI (Cesari et al. 2017b; Fried et al. 2011).

In the mediation between frailty and disability, an important role is also played by sarcopenia, intended as the loss of muscle lean mass and muscle strength (Cruz-Jentoft et al. 2019). Similar to frailty, there is large discussion about definition and measurement of sarcopenia (Cesari et al. 2016b). Nevertheless, there is a growing consensus in the literature about the importance of introducing the evaluation of the skeletal muscle in the clinical routine in order to identify (and eventually manage) individual exposed to an increased risk of mobility and physical disability.

Irrespective of the debate around defining and measuring it, that is outside the aims of this chapter, sarcopenia may represent the organ-specific pathophysiological background of the progressive reduction of the physical domain of intrinsic capacity, thus potentially influencing the ability to reach and maintain the full functional ability of the individual (Cesari et al. 2016b).

Sarcopenia may represent a novel clinical condition (a specific ICD10 is today available for it), legitimately entering in the computation of the multimorbidity construct, and have the role of biological substratum for the fragilization of the aging individual (Cesari et al. 2016b).

1.5 Frailty Epidemiology

Given the heterogeneous way of measuring frailty, it is clear that every estimate of its prevalence in the population might become easily arguable or (at best) provide a very partial vision of the phenomenon. Nevertheless, several studies have tried to estimate how frail some populations are across settings, countries, and regions.

In a systematic review and meta-analysis based on 21 studies (Collard et al. 2012), the prevalence of frailty ranges between 4.0% and 59.1%. The estimates were significantly lower when the analysis was restricted only to those studies adopting the frailty phenotype. When different subgroups were examined, women showed a substantially higher prevalence of frailty compared to men. As expected, prevalence increased with age, being the highest in subjects ≥ 85 years (Collard et al. 2012). These data are consistent with those coming from the Survey of Health, Aging and Retirement in Europe (SHARE) project and also further verified in other cohorts coming from the Asian countries (Cesari et al. 2016c).

Socio-economic factors are also closely related to frailty prevalence (Poli et al. 2017; Bandeen-Roche et al. 2015). Several studies have demonstrated that socially and/or economically disadvantaged persons present particularly high prevalence of frailty.

Last but not least, it is important to consider the weight of clinical conditions in the prevalence of frailty. It is obvious that a sicker person is more likely to appear frailty, independently of the adopted instrument to assess it. What is here meant is that frailty prevalence may be very different across clinical settings (Bandeen-Roche et al. 2015; Searle et al. 2018).

1.6 The Geriatric Approach to Frailty

In a recent document published by the British Geriatrics Society (British Geriatrics Society 2017), frailty is described as the condition defining individuals in the need of an adapted/integrated care approach based on the comprehensive geriatric assessment. The recommendations do not indicate a single tool to screen frailty (thus implicitly allowing a non-standardization of the results). The intervention offered to the individuals screening positive to frailty is prioritized over the eventual heterogeneity of the screening results. The document explains that, once the frail status of the individual is detected, the possible causes should be explored via a comprehensive geriatric assessment conducted by a multidisciplinary team, pursuing the final aim of designing a person-tailored intervention.

A change of paradigms for moving from the traditional disease-based approach towards a person-tailored model based on the comprehensive assessment of the aging individual is necessary. Today, the reshaping of our healthcare and clinical models is even solicited by the WHO, which recognize the inadequacy of available systems and evokes cornerstone messages of geriatric medicine (e.g., comprehensive assessment, focus on functions, evaluation of the environment, integration of care) (WHO 2015, 2017). In this context, shifting the focus from the disease to frailty may imply more attention to those deficits that concur at the fragilization of the individual but are not (yet) nosologically recognized. It implies paying attention to those abnormalities that are often complained by the older person but find no solution in a system concentrated in the prescription of drugs.

This type of approach has been classically a prerogative of geriatric medicine (Cesari et al. 2016a, c). It is today necessary to train other health professionals at the key principles of geriatrics for two main reasons: (1) age-related conditions requiring pills of geriatric expertise are today burdening every clinical setting and specialty; (2) geriatricians are too few for taking charge of every individual older than 65 (or 70? or 75?...) years.

1.7 Conclusions

Frailty is a clinical condition characterized by an excessive vulnerability of the individual to endogenous and exogenous stressors. This status generates a high risk of developing negative health-related events. Although sharing some characteristics with conditions such as multimorbidity and disability, frailty should not be confused with them. Several tools exist to evaluate frailty, and the choice of the proper one should be driven by the decisional algorithm and intervention it is going to feed.

Our aging societies require a substantial revision of our models of care. Frailty may represent a condition able to lever these changes and introduce neglected aspects of old age (e.g., function, social issues, Ethics) in the traditional medicine (largely based on the obsolete concept of disease). Shifting to a construct as frailty to biologically define the perimeter of action for geriatric medicine will probably concur at modernizing the old way of practicing medicine.

References

Bandeen-Roche K, Seplaki CL, Huang J, Buta B, Kalyani RR, Varadhan R et al (2015) Frailty in older adults: a nationally representative profile in the United States. J Gerontol Ser A Biol Sci Med Sci 70:1427–1434. https://doi.org/10.1093/gerona/glv133

Barnett K, Mercer SW, Norbury M, Watt G, Wyke S, Guthrie B (2012) Epidemiology of multimorbidity and implications for health care, research, and medical education: a cross-sectional study. Lancet 380:37–43. https://doi.org/10.1016/S0140-6736(12)60240-2

British Geriatrics Society (2017) Royal college of general practitioners and age UK. Fit for Frailty—Consensus Best Practice Guidance for the care of older people living with frailty in community and outpatient settings: a report from the British Geriatrics Society

Buta BJ, Walston JD, Godino JG, Park M, Kalyani RR, Xue Q-L et al (2016) Frailty assessment instruments: systematic characterization of the uses and contexts of highly-cited instruments. Ageing Res Rev 26:53–61. https://doi.org/10.1016/j.arr.2015.12.003

Castro HHG, Alencar AP, Benseor IM, Lotufo PA, Goulart AC (2017) Multimorbidities are associated to lower survival in Ischaemic stroke: results from a Brazilian stroke cohort (EMMA Study). Cerebrovasc Dis 44:232–239. https://doi.org/10.1159/000479827

Cesari M, Calvani R, Marzetti E (2017a) Frailty in older persons. Clin Geriatr Med 33:293–303. https://doi.org/10.1016/j.cger.2017.02.002

Cesari M, Marzetti E, Thiem U, Pérez-Zepeda MU, Abellan Van Kan G, Landi F et al (2016) The geriatric management of frailty as paradigm of "The end of the disease". Eur J Intern Med 31:11–14. https://doi.org/10.1016/j.ejim.2016.03.005

Cesari M, Nobili A, Vitale G (2016b) Frailty and sarcopenia: From theory to clinical implementation and public health relevance. Eur J Intern Med 35:1–9. https://doi.org/10.1016/j.ejim.2016.07.021

Cesari M, Pérez-Zepeda MU, Marzetti E (2017b) Frailty and multimorbidity: different ways of thinking about geriatrics. J Am Med Dir Assoc 18:361–364. https://doi.org/10.1016/j.jamda.2016.12.086

Cesari M, Prince M, Thiyagarajan JA, De Carvalho IA, Bernabei R, Chan P et al (2016c) Frailty: an emerging public health priority. J Am Med Dir Assoc 17:188–192. https://doi.org/10.1016/j.jamda.2015.12.016

Collard RM, Boter H, Schoevers RA, Oude Voshaar RC (2012) Prevalence of frailty in community-dwelling older persons: a systematic review. J Am Geriatr Soc 60:1487–1492. https://doi.org/10.1111/j.1532-5415.2012.04054.x

Cruz-Jentoft AJ, Bahat G, Bauer J, Boirie Y, Bruyère O, Cederholm T et al (2019) Sarcopenia: revised European consensus on definition and diagnosis. Age Ageing 48:16–31. https://doi.org/10.1093/ageing/afy169

Fraccaro P, Kontopantelis E, Sperrin M, Peek N, Mallen C, Urban P et al (2016) Predicting mortality from change-over-time in the Charlson Comorbidity Index: a retrospective cohort study in a data-intensive UK health system. Medicine (Baltimore) 95:e4973. https://doi.org/10.1097/MD.0000000000004973

Fried LP, Ferrucci L, Darer J, Williamson JD, Anderson G (2011) Untangling the concepts of disability, frailty, and comorbidity: implications for improved targeting and care. J Gerontol Ser A Biol Sci Med Sci 59:M255–M263. https://doi.org/10.1093/gerona/59.3.m255

Fried LP, Tangen CM, Walston J, Newman AB, Hirsch C, Gottdiener J et al (2001) Frailty in older adults: evidence for a phenotype. J Gerontol A Biol Sci Med Sci 56:M146–M156

Mannucci PM, Nobili A (2014) Multimorbidity and polypharmacy in the elderly: lessons from REPOSI. Intern Emerg Med 9:723–734. https://doi.org/10.1007/s11739-014-1124-1

Masnoon N, Shakib S, Kalisch-Ellett L, Caughey GE (2017) What is polypharmacy? A systematic review of definitions. BMC Geriatr 17:230. https://doi.org/10.1186/s12877-017-0621-2

Mitnitski AB, Mogilner AJ, Rockwood K (2001) Accumulation of deficits as a proxy measure of aging. ScientificWorldJournal 1:323–336. https://doi.org/10.1100/tsw.2001.58

Morley JE, Vellas B, van Kan GA, Anker SD, Bauer JM, Bernabei R et al (2013) Frailty consensus: a call to action. J Am Med Dir Assoc 14:392–397. https://doi.org/10.1016/j.jamda.2013.03.022

Muth C, Blom JW, Smith SM, Johnell K, Gonzalez-Gonzalez AI, Nguyen TS et al (2019) Evidence supporting the best clinical management of patients with multimorbidity and polypharmacy: a systematic guideline review and expert consensus. J Intern Med 285:272–288. https://doi.org/10.1111/joim.12842

National Institute for Health and Care Excellence (2017) Multimorbidity Overview

Payne RA (2016) The epidemiology of polypharmacy. Clin Med (Northfield Il) 16:465–469. https://doi.org/10.7861/clinmedicine.16-5-465

Poli S, Cella A, Puntoni M, Musacchio C, Pomata M, Torriglia D et al (2017) Frailty is associated with socioeconomic and lifestyle factors in community-dwelling older subjects. Aging Clin Exp Res 29:721–728. https://doi.org/10.1007/s40520-016-0623-5

Searle SD, Rockwood K (2018) What proportion of older adults in hospital are frail? Lancet 391:1751–1752. https://doi.org/10.1016/S0140-6736(18)30907-3

Tinetti ME, Fried T (2004) The end of the disease era. Am J Med 116:179–185

United Nations (2015) Department of Economic and Social Affairs, Population Division. World Population Ageing (ST/ESA/SER.A/390). 2015

Vetrano DL, Palmer K, Marengoni A, Marzetti E, Lattanzio F, Roller-Wirnsberger R et al (2018) Frailty and multimorbidity: a systematic review and meta-analysis. J Gerontol A Biol Sci Med Sci. https://doi.org/10.1093/gerona/gly110

WHO (2015) WHO World report on ageing and health 2015. World Health Organization. https://doi.org/10.1016/j.jmgm.2016.10.012

WHO (2017) Integrated care for older people : recommendations on interventions to manage declining physical and mental capacities in older people at community level

2 Tools for Assessing Frailty in Older People: General Concepts

Finbarr C. Martin and Aisling M. O'Halloran

Abstract

The general notion of frailty is widely understood to be a state of increased vulnerability to stressors, following age-related declines in function and reserves across multiple physiological systems. Frailty is clinically characterised by slower and/or incomplete recovery from stressors such as infection, injury, surgery or psychosocial distress. There is however no consensus on a single operational definition. Numerous assessment tools and scores are promoted to detect or measure frailty but two have widest research background and acceptance, the Frailty Phenotype and the deficit based Frailty Index. We describe these and other approaches in the context of a description of the psychometric properties, types of scaling, uses and misuses of assessment tools. We advocate the choice of an appropriate measurement tool be based on the population characteristics and the purpose for which it is to be used and illustrate how an understanding of the properties of different tools helps to inform this choice.

Keywords

Frailty · Prevalence · Epidemiology · Accuracy · Prognosis · Fried · Rockwood · Diagnosis

2.1 What Is Frailty? Introduction to the Concept

The broad consensus about the notion of frailty is of a person (more likely an older person) at heightened vulnerability to adverse health status change, in response to a stressor challenge such as infection, injury, surgery or psychosocial distress. This followed several decades of largely descriptive reports identifying the nature and scale of variation in the health of people of similar age. Isaacs, the UK based geriatrician who coined the term geriatric giants for the syndromes we now refer to as falls, incontinence, delirium or dementia, immobility and reduced functional ability (Isaacs 1980) described these as pre-death events related to widespread advanced ageing changes occurring often without clear disease correlates.

Rowe and Kahn's seminal paper published over 30 years ago (Rowe and Khan 1987) described the broad range of ageing-related physiological heterogeneity and distinguished

F. C. Martin · A. M. O'Halloran (✉)
The Irish Longitudinal Study on Ageing (TILDA), Trinity College Dublin, Dublin, Ireland
e-mail: AIOHALLO@tcd.ie

N. Veronese (ed.), *Frailty and Cardiovascular Diseases*, Advances in Experimental Medicine and Biology 1216, https://doi.org/10.1007/978-3-030-33330-0_2

usual from successful aging, where these changes were less marked and attributed much of this to favourable lifestyle factors. Chronological age, years lived, is therefore an inadequate predictor for the extent of ageing-related changes accumulated during these years but they do inevitably accumulate.

The idea of heighted vulnerability mentioned above has two aspects. Firstly, it suggests greater vulnerability than would have typically existed when the person was younger. With this meaning, although there remains some uncertainty as to whether frailty is inevitable, potentially all older people develop this heightened vulnerability if they live into advanced old age. Secondly, it implies that some older person's vulnerability is greater than others of the same age and this suggests the potential for stratifying populations for targeted interventions if this vulnerability can be measured. Although age-related changes gradually progress, multifactorial interventions targeted to improving and maintaining nutrition, physical activity and social engagement may enable frailty to reverse (Gill et al. 2006; Ng et al. 2015; Luger et al. 2016).

Frailty has been consistently shown to be a risk factor for falls, disability, cognitive impairment, dementia, hospital admission, increased length of hospital stay, post-operative complications, long-term residential care and mortality (Clegg et al. 2013; Fried et al. 2004; Lin et al. 2016; Hubbard and Story 2014; Cesari et al. 2016; Sirven and Rapp 2017; Rose et al. 2014; Roe et al. 2017).

The explanation for the vulnerability has been extensively researched (Walston et al. 2006; Clegg et al. 2013). An age-associated pro-inflammatory state, hormonal changes, reduced mitochondrial function, nutritional and other factors may all be involved, producing change at the cellular and organ-system level with impaired homeostatic responses being common manifestations (Puts et al. 2005; Leng et al. 2007). Cognitive changes and psycho-social factors are important modifiers of the impact of stressors but are not always included in the concept (or operationalisations) of frailty. An international consensus characterised "cognitive frailty" as a heterogeneous clinical state with both physical frailty and reduced cognitive reserves (Dartigues and Amieva 2014).

2.1.1 How Is Frailty Diagnosed and Measured?

There are plenty of assessment tools to screen for, diagnose or measure the severity of frailty, many of which have not been shown to be valid *and* reliable *and* diagnostically accurate *and* to have good predictive ability (Apóstolo et al. 2017). Predictiveness of adverse health outcomes is intrinsic to the notion and therefore a key aspect of validity. The variety of measurement approaches reflects the lack of consensus on what should be regarded as the necessary domains or parameters to be included (Rodríguez-Mañas et al. 2012). Nevertheless, a consensus has emerged around two operational approaches: the frailty phenotype and the deficit accumulation approach, and in judging all the main assessment tools against the specific criteria suggested by Clegg et al. (2013), these were considered the most robust (Dent et al. 2016).

The criteria were:

- ability to reliably predict adverse clinical outcomes
- an ability to reliably predict patient response to potential therapies
- be supported by a biological causative theory
- be simple to apply

The "Fried" phenotype approach (Fried et al. 2001) was derived and validated from the longitudinal US based Cardiovascular Health Study of 5,317 men and women aged 65 years and older on the basis of prediction of adverse outcomes over several subsequent years. The key point is that the variables collected were based on the proposition that certain parameters represented evidence of clinically relevant reduced physiological function. The five that emerged from analysis were unintentional weight loss, self reported fatigue and diminished physical activity, and measured impairment (comparative to age-standardised norms) of grip strength and gait speed. Whilst these clinical features often associated with diseases, they are nosologically distinct. The definition of frailty (and the intermediate/prodromal/subclincal state of pre-frailty) are based on the presence of three (or one or two) of these 5 variables being outside a normative range.

This phenotypic approach lends itself to the proposition that frailty is a syndrome with underlying physiological and metabolic changes, which may be inter-related and which are responsible for driving progressive physical and/or cognitive impairments through to loss of functional capacity, often helped on the way by acute or chronic disease or injury. This was anticipated a few years earlier in a slightly more elaborate definition of frailty than the broad idea mentioned above: *"a condition or syndrome which results from a multi-system reduction in reserve capacity to the extent that a number of physiological systems are close to, or past the threshold of symptomatic failure. As a result the frail person is at increased risk of disability or death from minor external stresses."* (Campbell and Buckner 1997).

The deficit accumulation approach operationalises frailty as a collection of symptoms, health behaviours, clinical signs, diagnoses, and functional limitations, each of which is not rare, increases in prevalence with age whilst not becoming universal and plausibly contribute to poorer health states. (Rockwood and Mitnitski 2007) Thus grey hair is excluded but anaemia and memory problems are included. The metric for each variable is dichotomized (or occasionally trichotomised) into a deficit (e.g. visual loss or high blood pressure or excess alcohol intake) being present or absent. Then the number of deficits present is divided by the total number assessed and the result expressed as a fraction of one. This number is the Frailty Index. It has a theoretical score range from 0 to 1.0 but extensive data has demonstrated that scores above 0.7 are very unusual, being incompatible with life (Rockwood and Mitnitski 2006; Bennett et al. 2013).

The variables can be collected from a comprehensive multidimensional (geriatric) assessment, as long as this covers a wide range of domains and includes upwards of 30+ variables. The Frailty Index (FI) can also be derived from routinely collected clinical data as in a primary care clinical record (Clegg et al. 2016) or an epidemiological survey dataset (Romero-Ortuno et al. 2010). This approach is also validated by its ability to identify people at higher risk of adverse health outcomes and mortality, and has subsequently been shown to be robust in this ability across many clinical and population cohorts in many countries, using a variety of deficits in the frailty indices.

These two approaches appear quite distinct but it has been suggested that the underlying pathophysiological factors may not be distinct as the deficits reflect underlying ubiquitous age related cellular changes (Howlett and Rockwood 2013) . Furthermore there is significant overlap in the distribution of the FI scores and the robust/pre-frail/frail categorisations from the Fried phenotype in community and clinical populations (Rockwood and Mitnitski 2007). Frailty measured with either approach is more prevalent in the oldest old and in those with the greatest burden of co-morbidity, chronic disease and disability but frailty and summative morbidity or disability scores do not map exactly within the older population. This is consistent with the notion that frailty is both a conceptually and epidemiologically distinct entity (Fried et al. 2004) .

The Fried phenotype assessment requires some simple equipment and normative data. Constructing a frailty index requires substantial clinical information and in a new patient, a comprehensive geriatric assessment.

Many other frailty tools are simpler and may be suitable for some purposes, including screening. Screening tools ranging from simple performance measures such as gait speed to composite clinical judgements (Rockwood et al. 2005) have been developed to detect frail individuals in community dwelling populations and clinical settings (Apóstolo et al. 2017). Whilst most are insufficient by the criteria described earlier for a definitive diagnosis of frailty, they may nevertheless be useful and more feasible for some purposes. Their utility depends on what the information is to be used for (Martin and Brighton 2008).

2.2 The Purposes of Detecting and Measuring Frailty

Could the recognition of frailty offer added value in the management of patients with acute illness or chronic conditions? It is recognised that disease-specific factors do not fully explain well-being and quality of life (Yohannes et al. 1998) and frailty may contribute independently of diseases severity. Comprehensive geriatric assessment already encompasses an approach which combines disease specific and non-specific aspects to the assessment and treatment of older people. Frailty recognition and management would be a refinement of this approach. In the surgical setting, the ability to improve prediction of post-operative functional recovery from cardiac surgery would provide added information for patients and inform clinical decisions, as disease based predictive models are far from perfect (Hamel et al. 2005).

Although there are good reasons for achieving agreement on the standardised tools described above to diagnose frailty, the choice of assessment will also depend upon the context and the purpose. What is the question being asked and what are the resources available—time, skill, people, and equipment? Here we summarise the range of contexts in which the addition of frailty assessment could help.

2.2.1 Clinical Decision Making About Individual Patients

- Suitability for medical or surgical treatments in which the potential benefits, risks and burdens will be impacted by the degree of frailty, in addition to the severity of the index condition being considered.
- Identifying how best to optimise physiological function (reduce vulnerability) such as respiration function or strength to achieve better outcomes from an acute medical event, injury or medical procedure.
- Monitoring clinical progress following a treatment programme.

2.2.2 Managing a Clinical Care Pathway

- Risk stratification (including screening) to identify people among a relatively low risk population who are likely to benefit from
  - a more detailed assessment, which may be broader and deeper in scope (and thus require more resources)
  - a different treatment pathway.
- To describe the casemix of patients referred to or using a service
  - In order to design a service in terms of the resources and skills needed
  - To estimate (changing) need over time.

2.2.3 Research

- To describe a research patient population to better understand the generalizability of the benefits, risks and burden associated with a treatment being evaluated.

Clearly, the types of assessment for screening, case finding, diagnosis, targeting etc. may need tools with different properties.

2.3 Properties of Assessment Tools

Tools may or may not do exactly as you would expect from the name given by their authors. The performance of tools can be systematically described, according to the qualities explained in Table 2.1.

These properties and how to assess and report them have been described in the COSMIN checklist, which also considers cross cultural validity, measurement error incorporating

Table 2.1 Properties of assessment tools in health and social care

Property	Explanation
Validity	Does the tool do what it says that it does?
Face	Does it seem to be about the issue of interest?
Content	The degree which the items match some objective criterion
Construct	Does the tool include the attributes understood to make up the health outcome or process being measured (e.g. Frailty) and in appropriate relative proportion
Predictive	Does the tool result predict subsequent events as expected
Concurrent	Does the tool result match that of an alternative, preferably well established, tool which addresses the same issue
Reliability	Does the tool give consistent results?
Test-retest	Does the tool produce consistent results when tested repeatedly in a stable situation
Inter-rater	Do different raters obtain consistent results when assessing the same person in the same context
Format	Does the tool behave the same in a variety of alternative formats, such as self-completion, face to face, by telephone, proxy scoring
Internal consistency	Do items in the tool behave in a consistent way relative to each other: internal agreement between parts of the whole tool
Responsiveness	Does the tool detect change when this is evident by some other appraisal
Feasibility	Can it be used in the real clinical situation it is intended for? This includes resource requirements, time, skill, and convenience
Acceptability	Is the experience of the tested participants satisfactory?

This is adapted from:
Springer International Publishing AG 2018
Series: Practical Issues in Geriatrics
Book title: Comprehensive Geriatric Assessment
Alberto Pilotto and Finbarr C Martin (eds)
2018
Chapter and Table author: Finbarr C Martin
Table 3.1 Properties of assessment tools in health and social care

standard error of measurement, smallest detectable change and limits of agreement (Mokkink et al. 2010).

2.3.1 Scaling

How the findings of the assessment are represented has an important impact on several of these qualities. Types of scaling are:

Categorical: this is a scale with two or more distinct descriptors without necessarily having any ordering or quantitative relationship to each other. Examples include ethnic group or sex. Some frailty tools produce a categorical result, such as frail or prefrail or robust (Fried phenotype) but these categories are based on specific numeric measures and there is an implicit ordering of the underlying construct defining the categories.

Ordinal: in these scales, numbers are used as labels which do have an intended ordering, but the basis of the numbers is really categorical. For example, the Edmonton Frail Scale (EFS) (Rolfson et al. 2006) ascribes numbers to the presence or absence of things such as polypharmacy or low mood. Therefore, the same numeric score can be obtained in a variety of ways. Two individuals with the same score may have quite different features. A higher score depicts more frailty associated characteristics but there is no consistent difference in the amount of frailty with each additional score from 0 to 2 etc. up to the maximum frailty score of 17. But that does not necessarily matter if when tested the predictiveness of a score is fairly consistent. It would matter however if the intention was to apply a standard intervention based on the score regardless of the contributions of the underlying items. **Interval:** In these scales, the numbers are based on a consistent quantity of the entity being measured, such as temperature. Some frailty associated performance measures, such as gait speed expressed in metres per second could be regarded as interval scales but usually there is a selected cut-point which is used to categorise. Since there is no underlying single biomarker which constitutes frailty, there is no pure frailty scale.

In the categorical and ordinal scales there is an implicit weighting applied to the items. So for example, fatigue and unintentional weight loss each provide one point towards the Fried categorisation but in what way are they actually equal in quantity? In the EFS, 0–2 points can be scored for functional ability but only 0–1 for continence. In most such weighted scales, there is no underlying theoretical rationale for the weighting but sometimes they arise from statistical modeling of predictiveness so are justified on this basis.

2.3.2 Screening, Case Finding and Rapid Assessment

There can be some confusion regarding these terms. All have a role in the context of frailty but in different contexts.

Screening is "*the process of identifying healthy people who may be at increased risk of disease or condition…*" (Public Health England 2013) or "Screening refers to the use of simple tests across an apparently healthy population in order to identify individuals who have risk factors or early stages of disease, but do not yet have symptoms" (WHO). These are slightly different definitions but the main point is that screening is not about making a diagnosis but identifying those with a higher probability of having or developing the problem. Criteria for a screening test include being reasonably cheap and acceptable with the acceptance that some who screen positive are false and some real positives are missed. Routine measurement of gait speed of all people who reach 70 years old could be an example, but would be justified only if it was followed by a more definitive assessment and offer of an intervention likely to improve future health outcomes.

Case finding is also about stratifying in a population but actively searching for the presence of the condition in individuals or groups who are suspected to be at risk. In this instance a group at risk might be older people presenting with a fall and the case finding would require an accepted diagnostic assessment such as the Frailty phenotype or Frailty Index.

As mentioned earlier there are many quicker and/or easier assessment approaches for frailty. A rapid assessment may be used to identify people likely to be frail (screening) and following this up with a more detailed assessment OR to assess some characteristics of a person who is likely to be frail in order to identify relevant clinical features relevant for risk prediction or treatment planning. In this case the important issue is the ability of the rapid assessment to identify those at greater risk, which can only be established empirically.

2.3.3 Clinical Prediction Tools

Tools and scales vary in their ability to discriminate, i.e. to detect an issue when it is present (or not) or predict that a specific clinical outcome or event will happen or not happen. The terms used to describe the properties of tools are set out in Table 2.2.

When a score on a scale is used to identify a "positive" prediction, there is a choice to be made about the most suitable cut point. This is usually done by plotting a receiver operating curve (ROC) to identify the optimum combination of sensitivity and specificity. A random

Table 2.2 Properties of predictive tools

Term	Explanation
Sensitivity	The hit rate: the proportion of real positives (with the issue, or who experience the clinical outcome of interest) who are correctly identified by a positive assessment
Specificity	The proportion of real negatives (those without the issue or who do not experience the outcome of interest) who are accurately identified or predicted by a negative assessment
accuracy	Correct identifications or predictions as a percentage of the total predictions made
Positive predictive value	Precision: the likelihood that a person identified as positive really has the issue or experiences the clinical outcome of interest
Negative predictive value	Precision: the likelihood that a person identified as negative really does not have the issue or experience the clinical outcome of interest

association of a positive test result and the clinical outcome produces a ROC area under the curve of 0.5. Total concordance would produce a value of 1.0. In general, a ROC value of about 0.8 or above is regarded as clinically useful. Clinical or epidemiological studies which demonstrate impressive associations between, for example, a combination of variables in a tool, and a clinical outcome do not necessarily make prediction tools which have clinical utility, but lower ROC values are certainly sufficient to demonstrate significant associations and this can be useful for risk stratification or better understanding of causal factors or case mix description.

For a prediction tool to be useful it must also be applicable to groups other than those involved with its initial development. However, even when validated in a new "remote" population, predictive values observed in one context do not apply universally. A key issue here is the effect of prevalence on predictiveness. Assuming the same sensitivity and specificity, the rarer the issue being predicted (e.g. occult disease or a specific clinical outcome) the more likely that a negative test is a true negative, but the likelihood that a positive result is a true positive becomes less. Thus clinical utility of a tool in one setting (e.g. a clinic with many frail persons) cannot be assumed to be as useful in another, such as a generally healthy community dwelling population. The threshold for defining frailty (or high risk) is likely also impacted by the exposure period - the time interval between assessment of risk and the outcome.

The demonstration that a clinical prediction tool is fit for purpose has several stages, and these are set out in the TRIPOD statement for reporting them (Collins et al. 2015). In addition it is important to establish if a tool with adequate predictive accuracy can lead to better outcomes and ultimately be incorporated into routine clinical practice. These stages are described briefly in Table 2.3.

2.4 Which Tool for Which Purpose?

Whereas some tools may be judged to be poor by their failure to attain the key qualities outlined earlier, caution should be applied before concluding that a good tool is suitable for any purpose. It depends on what the information is to be used for. There is a range of potential purposes and a range of contexts: these factors will influence which tools or assessment approach is suitable,

2.4.1 Screening

Since the usual purpose of a screening tool is simply and quickly to differentiate people into those with different likelihoods of being frail (or of being at risk of experiencing a poor outcome with a proposed treatment etc.), it should be short

Table 2.3 Stages in the creation of a useful clinical prediction tool

Stage	Explanation
Concept	– What is the tool to be used for, and in what context?
Development	– Which parameters should be considered for inclusion? Clinical and epidemiological data will inform this – Select variables which are feasible to measure and use in routine practice – Test the relationships between individual and combinations of these variables and the outcome of interest in existing or new longitudinal datasets – Design a scoring system and identify suitable cut-points based on ROC analysis
Validation	– Test whether the tool is better than usual clinical judgement: does it add value? – Test the reproducibility of discrimination in a remote cohort, e.g. a similar clinical group in a different hospital or community
Impact	– Test whether use of the tool results in better clinical outcomes or more efficient resource use
Implementation and spread	– Assess feasibility and user friendliness – The tool may need adaption in format and presentation for different settings, but changing variables or cut-points would require revalidation

and fairly sensitive in identifying those needing special attention, and specific, so as to avoid providing unneeded interventions to robust patients falsely classified as pre-frail or frail. Available instruments tend to have high sensitivity but limited specificity. Frailty screening instruments must also have good positive and negative predictive values, which are influenced by the prevalence of frailty. These will be the instruments most useful at population level. In the absence of a "gold standard", the instrument to screen and diagnose frailty should be chosen according to the characteristics of the population being studied, the aims of the assessment and the clinical context (Martin and Brighton 2008; Cesari et al. 2014).

A recent umbrella review analysed the findings of five systematic reviews inclusive of 227,381 participants (Apóstolo et al. 2017). This looked at the qualities of 26 questionnaires and brief assessments and eight frailty indicators, most of which had been evaluated in use with community-dwelling older people, including studies in which the frailty prevalence was lower than in older clinical populations. The reviews differed in their focus including the predictive accuracy for identifying frailty and/or for predicting adverse outcomes.

Gait speed showed high sensitivity, but only moderate specificity, and excellent predictive ability for future disability in activities of daily living, in a community population over longish time periods. The Timed-up-and-go test (Podsiadlo and Richardson 1991) and PRISMA 7 (preferred reporting items for systematic reviews and meta-analyses) (Raiche et al. 2008) have high sensitivity and moderate specificity for identifying frailty. The Tilburg Frailty Indicator (Gobbens et al. 2010) is a reliable and accurate predictive tool for clinical outcomes, although it does not provide a definitive frailty diagnosis.

2.4.2 Clinical Decision Making

In clinical populations such as in surgery pre-assessment clinic, the choice may not necessarily be to identify frailty definitively but to stratify by risk and/or identify potentially modifiable factors. These might include medical conditions such as under treated airways disease or unrecognized ischaemic heart disease but also frailty related factors such as cognitive impairment as a risk factor for delirium or fatigue suggesting poor endurance and therefore risk of poor functional recovery. The well developed Multidimensional Prognostic Index predicts worse clinical trajectories for patients with heart failure (Pilotto et al. 2010) and identifies risk levels for a variety of clinical populations including those undergoing Transcatheter Aortic Valve Implantation (TAVI) (Bureau et al. 2017).

Although it is a large step to translate prediction from large datasets which works epidemiologically to the precision needed in clinical practice, the FI has superior prediction of functional recovery and return home after hip fractures than the best disease-specific score (Krishnan et al. 2014). Generally however, frailty risk scores can identify those at higher risk but more detailed assessment is necessary to inform the balance of benefit, risk and burden for the individual patient.

2.4.3 Planning Clinical Services

For planning health services and deciding in broad terms where and for whom to apply health preventative interventions, the larger population predictive ability may suffice.

Aguayo et al. (2017) assessed the performance of 35 frailty scores or indicators, 23 of which showed a significant relationship with longer term incident cardiovascular events, with hazard ratios adjusted for sex between 1.2 and 16.5. These associations remained significant and sizeable for the majority after adjustment for other factors. This highlights the need to broaden the scope of risk modification beyond the traditional risk factors

2.5 Future Developments

Living with frailty, according to any of the established criteria, or having reduced functional ability are predictive of functional decline (or death) after significant stressors such as surgical procedures. However, no frailty tool is a complete and satisfactory measure of the totality of the reserves of physiological or psychosocial attributes which, if further depleted, contribute to this reduced functional ability. There is however a further source of variability which may be complementary to frailty but even more elusive. This may be termed resilience, although so far no consensus has yet emerged on the exact nature or definition of this (Whitson et al. 2016). Here we use this term to describe the propensity for underlying physiological processes to recover from a stressor. Clearly a relatively greater ability to withstand an apparently similar sized stressor will render the outcome different for two individuals who seem similar at the outset.

One difficulty here is that we lack a generalizable measure of the magnitude of a stressor. Nevertheless, to illustrate the point, consider that an observational study of recovery from delirium induced by an acute illness reported no relationship between recovery and the severity of physical illness (admission APACHE II, APS, BISEP) or disability (Barthel Index) (Adamis et al. 2006). If we could measure the amount of cognitive reserve, and this was also similar, then we may conclude that their resilience differed. At present this is speculative and further study is warranted to establish whether adding resilience to the dataset along with frailty would improve predictive accuracy and therefore inform clinical decision making. Furthermore, we don't know if pre-habilitation can impact resilience as well as enhancing measurable reserves.

References

Adamis D, Treloar A, Martin FC, Macdonald AJ (2006) Recovery and outcome of delirium in elderly medical inpatients. Arch Gerontol Geriatr 43(2):289–298

Apóstolo J, Cooke R, Bobrowicz-Campos E, Santana S, Marcucci M, Cano S et al (2017) Predicting risk and outcomes for frail older adults: an umbrella review of frailty screening tools. JBI Database Syst Rev Implement Rep 15:1154–1208

Aguayo G, Donneau A, Vaillan M, Schritz A, Franco O, Stranges S et al (2017) Agreement between 35 published frailty scores in the general population. Am J Epidemiol 186(4):420–434

Bennett S, Song X, Mitnitski A, Rockwood K (2013) A limit to frailty in very old, community-dwelling people: a secondary analysis of the Chinese longitudinal health and longevity study. Age Ageing 42:372–377

Bureau ML, Liuu E, Christiaens L, Pilotto A, Mergy J, Bellarbre F et al (2017) MPI AGE Project Investigators. Using a multidimensional prognostic index (MPI) based on comprehensive geriatric assessment (CGA) to predict mortality in elderly undergoing transcatheter aortic valve implantation. Int J Cardiol

236:381–386. https://doi.org/10.1016/j.ijcard.2017.02.048

Campbell AJ, Buckner DM (1997) Unstable disability and the fluctuations of frailty. Age Ageing 26(4):315–318

Cesari M, Gambassi G, van Kan GA, Vellas B (2014) Age Ageing 43(1):10–12. https://doi.org/10.1093/ageing/aft160

Cesari M, Prince M, Thiyagarajan JA, De Carvalho IA, Bernabei R, Chan P et al (2016) Frailty: an emerging public health priority. J Am Med Dir Assoc 17 (3):188–192

Clegg A, Young J, Iliffe S, Rikkert MO, Rockwood K (2013) Frailty in elderly people. Lancet 381:752–762

Clegg A, Bates C, Young J, Teale E, Parry J (2016) Development and validation of an electronic frailty index using routine primary care electronic health record data. Age Ageing 45(3):353–360. https://doi.org/10.1093/ageing/afw039

Collins CS, Reitsma JB, Altman DG, Moons KG (2015) Transparent reporting of a multivariable prediction model for individual prognosis or diagnosis (TRIPOD): the TRIPOD statement. Available via http://www.equator-network.org/reporting-guidelines/tripod-statement/ Accessed 30 Mar 2019

Dartigues JF, Amieva H (2014) Cognitive frailty: rational and definition from an (I.a.N.a./i.a.g.g.) international consensus group. J Nutr Health Aging 18:95. https://doi.org/10.1007/s12603-013-0437-5

Dent E, Kowal P, Hoogendijk EO (2016) Frailty measurement in research and clinical practice: a review. Eur J Int Med 31:3–10

Fried LP, Tangen CM, Walston J, Newman AB, Hirsch C, Gottdiener J et al for the Cardiovascular Health Study Collaborative Research Group (2001) Frailty in older adults: Evidence for a phenotype. J Gerontol A Biol Sci Med Sci 56: M146–M156

Fried LP, Ferrucci L, Darer J, Williamson JD, Anderson G (2004) Untangling the concepts of disability, frailty, and comorbidity: implications for improved targeting and care. J Gerontol A Biol Sci Med Sci 59(3):255–263

Gill TM, Gahbauer EA, Allore HG, Han L (2006) Transitions between frailty states among community-living older persons. Arch Intern Med 166(4):418–423

Gobbens RJ, van Assen MA, Luijkx KG, Wijnen-Sponselee MT Schols JM (2010) The tilburg frailty indicator: psychometric properties. JAMDA 11 (5):344–355

Hamel MB, Henderson WG, Khuri SF, Daley J (2005) Surgical outcomes for patients aged 80 and older: morbidity and mortality from major noncardiac surgery. J Am Geriatr Soc 53:424–429

Howlett S, Rockwood K (2013) New horizons in frailty: ageing and the deficit-scaling problem. Age Ageing 42 (4):416–423. https://doi.org/10.1093/ageing/aft059

Hubbard RE, Story DA (2014) Patient frailty: the elephant in the operating room. Anaesthesia 69(Suppl 1):26–34

Isaacs B (1980) The challenge of geriatric medicine. Oxford University Press, Oxford

Krishnan M, Beck S, Havelock W, Eeles E, Hubbard RE, Johansen A (2014) Predicting outcome after hip fracture: using a frailty index to integrate comprehensive geriatric assessment results. Age Ageing 43 (1):122–126

Leng SX, Xue QL, Tian J, Walston JD, Fried LP (2007) Inflammation and frailty in older women. J Am Geriatr Soc 55(6):864–871

Lin HS, Watts JN, Peel NM, Hubbard RE (2016) Frailty and post-operative outcomes in older surgical patients: a systematic review. BMC Geriatr 16(1):157

Luger, Dorner TE, Haider S Kapan A, Lackinger C, Schindler K (2016) Effects of a home-based and volunteer-administered physical training, nutritional, and social support program on malnutrition and frailty in older persons: a randomized controlled trial. J Am Med Dir Assoc 17:671.e9–671.e16

Martin FC, Brighton P (2008) Frailty: different tools for different purposes? Age Ageing 37:129–131. https://doi.org/10.1093/ageing/afn011

Mokkink LB, Terwee CB, Patrick DL, Alonso J, Stratford PW, Knol DL, Bouter LM, de Vet HCW (2010) The COSMIN checklist for assessing the methodological quality of studies on measurement properties of health status measurement instruments: an international Delphi study. Qual Life Res 19(4):539–549

Ng TP, Feng L, Nyunt MS, Feng L, Niti M, Tan BY et al (2015) Nutritional, physical, cognitive, and combination interventions and frailty reversal among older adults: a randomized controlled trial. Am J Med 128:1225–1236

Pilotto A, Addante F, Franceschi M, LeandromG, Rengo G, D'Ambrosio LP et al (2010) Multidimensional Prognostic Index based on a comprehensive geriatric assessment predicts short-term mortality in older patients with hert failure. Circ Heart Fail 3:191–199

Podsiadlo D, Richardson S (1991) The timed "Up & Go": a test of basic functional mobility for frail elderly persons. J Am Geriatr Soc 39:142–148

Public Health England (2013) NHS population screening explained. Available via https://www.gov.uk/guidance/nhs-population-screening-explained). Accessed 21 Mar 2019

Puts MTE, Visser M, Twisk JWR, Deeg DJH, Lips P (2005) Endocrine and inflammatory markers as predictors of frailty. Clin Endocrinol 63:403–411

Raiche M, Hebert R, Dubois MF (2008) PRISMA-7: a case-finding tool to identify older adults with moderate to severe disabilities. Arch Gerontol Geriatr 47 (1):9–18

Rockwood K, Mitnitski A (2006) Limits to deficit accumulation in elderly people. Mech Ageing Dev 127:494–496

Rockwood K, Mitnitski A (2007) Frailty in relation to the accumulation of deficits. J Gerontol A Biol Sci Med Sci 62(7):722–727

Rockwood K, Song X, MacKnight C, Bergman H, Hogan DB, McDowell I et al (2005) A global clinical measure of fitness and frailty in elderly people. CMAJ 173:489–495. https://doi.org/10.1503/cmaj.050051

Rodríguez-Mañas L, Féart C, Mann G, Viña J, Chatterji S, Chodzko-Zajko W, Vega E (2012) Searching for an operational definition of frailty: A Delphi method based consensus statement. The frailty operative definition-consensus conference project. J Gerontol A Biol Sci Med Sci 68(1): 62–67. https://doi.org/10.1093/gerona/gls119

Roe L, Normand C, Wren MA, Browne J, O'Halloran AM (2017) The impact of frailty on healthcare utilisation in Ireland: evidence from the Irish longitudinal study on ageing. BMC Geriatr 17(1):203. https://doi.org/10.1186/s12877-017-0579-0

Rolfson DB, Majumdar SR, Tsuyuki RT, Adeel T, Rockwood K (2006) Validity and reliability of the Edmonton Frail Scale. Age Ageing 35(5):526–529. https://doi.org/10.1093/ageing/afl041

Romero-Ortuno R, Walsh C, Lawlor BA, Kenny RA (2010) A frailty instrument for primary care: findings from the survey of health, ageing and retirement in Europe (SHARE). BMC Geriatr 10:57

Rose M, Pan H, Levinson MR, Staples M (2014) Can frailty predict complicated care needs and length of stay? Intern Med J 44(8):800–805

Rowe JW, Khan RL (1987) Human ageing: usual and successful. Science 237:143–149

Sirven N, Rapp T (2017) The cost of frailty in France. Eur J Health Econ 18:243–253

Walston J, Hadley EC, Ferrucci L, Guralnik JM, Newman AB, Studenski SA et al (2006) Research agenda for frailty in older adults: toward a better understanding of physiology and etiology: summary from the American geriatrics Society/National Institute on Aging Research conference on frailty in older adults. J Am Geriatr Soc 54(6):991–1001

Whitson HE, Duan-Porter W, Schmader KE et al (2016) Physical resilience in older adults: systematic review and development of an emerging construct. J Gerontol A Biol Sci Med Sci 71(4):489–495. https://doi.org/10.1093/gerona/glv202

Yohannes AM, Roomi J, Waters K, Connolly MJ (1998) Quality of life in elderly patients with COPD: measurement and predictive factors. Respir Med 92(10):1231–1236

3 Epidemiology of Frailty in Older People

Sabine Rohrmann

Abstract

Frailty is a complex of symptoms that is characterized by impaired stress tolerance due to a decline in the functionality of different organs. Due to its multifactorial aetiology, several definitions and assessments of this symptom complex have been developed, of which the Fried Frailty Score (Phenotype Score) and the broader Frailty Index (Deficit Accumulation Index) are the most commonly used. The prevalence of frailty increases with age independently of the assessment instrument and ranges between 4 and 59% in community-dwelling elderly populations and is higher in women than in men. The actual prevalence rate in a population depends on the prevalence of chronic diseases including depression, nutritional status, and inherently socio-economic background and education. Frailty is, however, not a steady state and progression, but also reversion is common. Although numerous studies on the prevalence of frailty have been conducted, systematic assessments in different populations are rare, which reduces the comparability of results. Similarly heterogeneous, but less frequent are studies on the incidence and on trajectories and transitions of frailty, calling for further, more systematic studies on this topic.

Keywords

Epidemiology · Frailty · Community · Nursing home

3.1 Introduction

Frailty is a complex of symptoms that is characterized by impaired stress tolerance due to a decline in the functionality of different organs because of sarcopenia, nutritional deficiencies, hormonal changes, and increased inflammation (Collerton et al. 2012; Fried et al. 2001). Though not a disease in itself, it is associated with an increased risk of falls, disability, hospitalization, institutionalization, and finally mortality (Fried et al. 2001; Clegg et al. 2013).

There is no uniform definition of the frailty symptom complex. However, most studies are based on the definition introduced by Fried et al. (2001), which includes unintentional weight loss, self-reported exhaustion, poor grip strength, slow walking speed, or low physical activity (Fried et al. 2001). This model is also called the Phenotype Model (Li et al. 2017). Individuals are usually considered as frail if they meet at least 3 of the 5 criteria and as prefrail if they meet 1 or 2 of these criteria. This definition has a focus on

S. Rohrmann (✉)
Division of Chronic Disease Epidemiology, Epidemiology, Biostatistics and Prevention Institute (EBPI), University of Zurich, Hirschengraben 84, 8001 Zurich, Switzerland
e-mail: sabine.rohrmann@uzh.ch

N. Veronese (ed.), *Frailty and Cardiovascular Diseases*, Advances in Experimental Medicine and Biology 1216, https://doi.org/10.1007/978-3-030-33330-0_3

the physical aspects of frailty. A more complex score, the so-called Frailty Index (or Frailty Index of Deficit Accumulation), was established by Mitnitski et al. (2002) based on the proportion of 20 deficits observed in a structured clinical examination. These deficits include diseases, signs, symptoms, laboratory abnormalities, cognitive impairments, and disabilities in activities of daily living (Pena et al. 2014). Other definitions exist, but these two, the Fried Frailty Score and the Frailty Index, are most frequently used in studies.

3.2 Prevalence

The prevalence of frailty has been assessed in many studies worldwide, although most studies were conducted in Western countries.

One of the most comprehensive reviews on the epidemiology of frailty included 21 community-based studies with 61,500 persons 65+ years old (Collard et al. 2012). Overall, the prevalence of frailty varied from 4.0 to 59.1% with an overall weighted prevalence of frailty of 10.7% (95% confidence interval (CI) 10.5–10.9). Of the 21 studies included, 14 used the Fried Frailty Score (Fried et al. 2001). A difference in the prevalence of frailty between studies emerged when studies were stratified by the assessment for frailty (Collard et al. 2012). In studies that assessed physical frailty, using e.g. the Fried Frailty Score, the prevalence rate ranged between 4.0 and 17.0%, but between 4.2 and 59.1% in studies that used broad definitions or measurement instruments (covering physical, but also social and psychological aspects for frailty). The weighted prevalence rate was 9.9% for physical frailty (95% CI 9.6–10.2; based on 15 studies with 44,894 participants) and 13.6% for the broad phenotype of frailty (95% CI 13.2–14.0; based on 8 studies with 24,072 participants).

Another review explicitly included only studies that used the Fried Frailty Score to assess the prevalence of frailty in community-dwelling individuals 65 years of age and older (Choi et al. 2015). In the six studies included, the prevalence of frailty ranged between 4.9% in Taiwan and 27.3% in Spain. The Survey of Health, Aging and Retirement in Europe (SHARE; Santos-Eggimann et al. 2009) assessed frailty in a uniform way in Europe and still yielded vastly different prevalence rates across Europe. Generally, they observed a prevalence of 17%, with lows of 5.8% in Switzerland and 8.6% in Sweden and a high prevalence rate of 23% in Italy and 27.3% in Spain. The prevalence rates of pre-frailty were more comparable between the single countries with 46.5% in Switzerland, 45.3% in Sweden, 43.6% in Italy, and 50.9% in Spain.

3.2.1 Geographic Variation

There is some indication that the prevalence of frailty and the extent of frailty is higher in poorer countries than in more affluent ones. A secondary analysis of the SHARE survey, which included more than 35,000 participants at least 50 years old from 15 countries, observed a lower mean frailty index in higher-income countries than in lower-income countries (Theou et al. 2013). The overall mean frailty index was inversely correlated with both gross domestic product ($r = -0.79$; $P < 0.01$) and health expenditure ($r = -0.63$; $P < 0.05$). The prevalence of frailty was lower in higher-income countries compared with lower-income countries (16.1 vs. 27.6%; $P < 0.01$). Interestingly, survival in non-frail participants 2 years after baseline assessment was not associated with national income, but survival in frail people was significantly better in higher-income countries (Theou et al. 2013). One explanation for the higher prevalence of frailty in Southern compared with Northern countries participating in the SHARE study might be the lower rates of institutionalization of older disabled persons in southern countries, leading to a higher prevalence of frailty in community-based studies.

In a systematic review of 47 studies that included community-dwelling adults 60+ years old in low- and middle-income countries, the pooled prevalence rate of frailty was 17.4% (95% CI 14.4–20.7%) (Siriwardhana et al. 2018). This is higher than the overall weighted prevalence of frailty of 10.7% (95% CI 10.5–10.9) in 21 studies from high-income countries (Collard et al. 2012). The prevalence rates of frailty varied between 3.9% in China and 51.4% in Cuba; the prevalence of prefrailty ranged from 13.4% in Tanzania to 71.6% in Brazil (Siriwardhana et al. 2018). However, only one low-income country (Tanzania) and one low-middle income country were included in that analysis; all other studies were conducted in high-middle income countries. The prevalence of prefrailty was 49.3% (95% CI 46.4–52.2%) in low- and middle-income countries (Siriwardhana et al. 2018), which was also higher than the pooled rate of 41.6% (95% CI 41.2–42.0%) in high-income countries (Collard et al. 2012).

It is interesting to note that even studies conducted in the same country do not always provide similar estimates. The FRALLE survey, conducted in the Spanish city of Lleida, reported a frailty prevalence of 9.6% in participants 75 + years old (5.2% in men and 12.5% in women; Jurschik et al. 2012), but other Spanish studies provided prevalence rates ranging from 10.3 to 20.1% (see Jurschik et al. 2012). In the US, the prevalence reported was also very disparate, ranging from 6.9% in the study by Fried et al. (2001) to 19.5% in the study among Mexican-Americans (Ottenbacher et al. 2005). A study looking at racial differences in the US observed that 8.7% of African-American men and 15.0% of African-American women were frail compared with 4.6% and 6.8% of white men and women, respectively (Hirsch et al. 2006). In adjusted models, taking age, sex, comorbidity, and socioeconomic factors into account, non-obese African Americans had fourfold greater odds of frailty compared with whites. This study also noted that the increased odds of frailty associated with African-American race was less pronounced among those who were obese or disabled. This study shows that, although socio-economic factor might play an important role, there may be other factors that play a role in the development of frailty. Large ranges were also reported from low- and middle-income countries. A systematic review reported that the prevalence rate of frailty in community-dwelling older people ranged between 17 and 31% in Brazil, between 5 and 31% in China, and from 21 to 44% in Russia, with all studies using the Fried Frailty Score (Nguyen et al. 2015).

A Chinese study that included individuals of 60+ years used the physical frailty phenotype scale and reported a frailty prevalence of 7%, which ranged between 3.3 and 9.1% depending on the study region (Wu et al. 2018). It was higher in rural than in urban areas and, as other studies had shown before, frail individuals were more likely to have co-morbidities and functional limitations than non-frail individuals were.

3.3 Incidence

Incidence studies on frailty are rare; most studies only describe the prevalence in a certain population. In the Cardiovascular Health Study, which included 5,317 participants 65 years and older, the four-year incidence was 7.4% (Fried et al. 2001). In an analysis of the longitudinal Osteoarthritis Initiative (OAI) database with 4421 study participants, the incidence of frailty amounted to 12 (95% CI 10–14) participants per 1000 person-years (Shivappa et al. 2018). In an analysis of the *Progetto Veneto Anziani*, which included 1887 individuals older than 65 years of age and free of frailty at baseline, 21.9% had become frail after an observation period of 4.4 years (Trevisan et al. 2016). These results illustrate the problems with respect to information on frailty incidence from longitudinal studies. Even if numbers of incident frailty cases are reported, it is difficult to compute incidence rates due to the lack of information on person-time. Moreover, hardly any study used age-standardization to make studies comparable. This was illustrated in a systematic review by Galluzzo et al. (2018). Only 3 of the 6 studies included had the aim of estimating frailty incidence, with a wide age-range of participants. The incidence proportion ranged from 5% (follow-up 22.2 years; age $\geq$ 30 years) to 13% (follow-up 1 year, age $\geq$ 55 years). Looking only at studies that used the Fried Frailty Score and were conducted on relatively similar samples in terms of age, the incidence proportions ranged from 3.9% for a follow-up of about 3 years to about 8% over periods from 3.5 to 9.9 years. The highest incidence rate was observed in an Australian study that included remotely living aboriginal people. Participants were 45+ years old, and of those who were non-frail at the beginning of the study, 51.5% became frail during the 7-year follow-up period (Hyde et al. 2016).

3.4 Reasons for Differences in the Prevalence of Frailty Between Populations

3.4.1 Differences Due to Different Assessment Instruments

The definition of frailty varies from physical disability, impairment in basic or instrumental activities of daily living to an increased vulnerability to adverse outcomes. In a review, Buta et al. identified 67 frailty assessment instruments that were mentioned in scientific publication, of which nine were highly-cited (≥ 200 citations) (Buta et al. 2016). The Physical Frailty Phenotype, as introduced by Fried et al., was the most frequently used frailty assessment instrument in the research literature, followed by the Deficit Accumulation Index and the Vulnerable Elders Survey. The definition by Fried et al. focuses on a wasting syndrome, with weight loss and negative energy balance as important elements (Fried et al. 2001). Other instruments have emphasized a life course approach, taking into account mid- and early-life influences on late-life frailty. Cognitive and social factors for improving the prediction of frailty are a more recent research focus (Buta et al. 2016). For example, a US study among 6000 community-dwelling elderly adults (65–95 years old) showed that including cognitive impairment as a variable improved the predictive validity of the operational definition of frailty (Avila-Funes et al. 2009). Another study conducted among 744 70 + year old community-dwelling individuals concluded that slow gait speed, low physical activity, weight loss, and cognitive impairment were key indicators of frailty, but questioned the usefulness of self-reported exhaustion and muscle weakness (Rothman et al. 2008).

Collard et al. (2012) showed in their meta-analysis that the differences in frailty prevalence rates were less diverse when assessments based on the physical frailty definition were used compared with a broader definition that also covers social and psychosocial aspects. The smaller range of frailty rates in the first group of studies might imply more consensus in the definition of frailty between researchers or a more reliable definition. The advantage is a better comparability of studies. If a broad frailty definition is used, it appears to be very important to examine separately the different aspects within the respective frailty definition. This will provide more information about who needs special care in specific domains, but may also enhance the understanding and disentangling of underlying pathophysiological processes of frailty.

3.4.2 Differences Due to Different Operationalizations of the Single Components of the Instrument

The Fried Frailty Score basically assesses slow walking, weak grip strength, low physical activity, exhaustion, and weight loss (Fried et al. 2001). However, depending on the concrete assessment of these five variables, the prevalence rate might differ even though the same definition has been used. This has been studied and discussed in the SHARE study. Criteria used to define frailty in the SHARE study were not identical to those used in the Cardiovascular Health Study, except for weakness, and may be less specific, leading to higher estimates of the prevalence particularly for exhaustion, which was common in the SHARE population (Santos-Eggimann et al. 2009). In a follow-up on this issue, Romero-Ortuno showed in detail how the categorization of study participants changed depending on how the five variables of the Fried Frailty Score were defined (Romero-Ortuno 2013).

3.4.3 Differences Due to Different Settings

The prevalence rates differ substantially depending on the setting where they have been conducted. Prevalence rates are substantially lower among community-dwelling individuals compared with institutionalized individuals living, e.g., in nursing homes. The review by Nguyen revealed a prevalence of frailty of 49% in institutionalized older patients in Brazil and 32% in hospitalized older patients in India. The prevalence of frailty in outpatient clinics was 55–71% in Brazil and 28% in Peru (Nguyen et al. 2015). As mentioned above, this may also differ between countries or regions, depending, for example, on whether older people are more likely to stay at home or with family member rather than living at nursery homes. This leads to lower or higher proportions of frail elderly in the community-dwelling population (Theou et al. 2013).

3.5 Risk Factors

A systematic review evaluated factors that were either risk or protective factors for frailty (Feng et al. 2017). In total, 23 longitudinal studies with community-dwelling individuals 60+ years old were included. Statistically significant associations with frailty were observed for sociodemographic factors (7/7 studies; this included older age, ethnic background, neighbourhood, and access to private insurance or Medicare), physical factors (5/6 studies; obesity and activities of daily living functional status), biological factors (5/7 studies; serum uric acid), lifestyle factors (11/13 studies; higher Diet Quality Index International score, higher fruit/vegetable consumption and higher tertile of all measures of habitual dietary resveratrol exposure), and psychological factors (7/8 studies; depressive symptoms). Many more factors have been analysed in these studies, but most of them either did not turn out to be significantly associated with frailty or were examined in only a small number of studies (Feng et al. 2017). The study among Australian aboriginal people clearly supports a multifactorial aetiology, including on the one hand underlying chronic diseases and on the other hand psychosocial stressors (Hyde et al. 2016).

Age and sex seem to be clearly associated with frailty. In the meta-analysis by Collard et al., the prevalence increased with age and was higher in women (9.6%, 95% CI 9.2–10.0%) than in men (5.2%, 95% CI 4.9–5.5%) (Fried et al. 2001). In the SHARE survey, at all ages, the mean frailty index was greater in women than in men regardless of country. Every additional year of age was associated with a 3.5 and 2.8% higher mean frailty index in lower- and higher-income countries, respectively (Theou et al. 2013). The difference by sex and the increase with age are seen in high- (Collard et al. 2012) as well as in low- and middle-income countries (Siriwardhana et al. 2018). The prevalence of frailty is higher in women compared to men because women have lower average amounts of lean body mass and muscle strength (Fried et al. 2001).

A systematic review and meta-analysis by Verlaan et al. (2017) assessed the prevalence of malnutrition and frailty among community-dwelling elderly, the prevalence of frailty ranged between 0% (a study in Taiwan) and 36.6% (in a Lebanese study). Pooling data from ten studies using comparable assessment instruments, the authors observed that the prevalence of physical frailty was higher among those with less favourable nutritional status such that 68.0% were frail in the malnourished group, but only 11.9% in the well-nourished group (as assessed using the Mini-Nutritional Assessment) (Verlaan et al. 2017). However, vice versa, the association was less clear. A prevalence rate of malnutrition of 0.5% was observed in the robust group and of 8.4% in the frail group.

3.5.1 Frailty Progression

So far, only few studies examined the progression of frailty. Most studies are cross-sectional in nature and do not observe changes over time. However, frailty is not a steady state. In a follow-up of the SHARE study that included individuals 55+ years old, frailty worsened in 22.1% of the participants within two years after the first assessment, remained stable in 61.8% of the participants and improved in 16.1% (Etman et al. 2012). The risk of worsening increased with age and was statistically significantly higher in individuals 65+ years old at baseline assessment, in women and in individuals with low education. It is interesting that participants from Southern European countries (France, Italy and Greece) had an increased risk of worsening at an earlier age compared with those in Northern and middle European countries (Sweden, Denmark, Germany, the Netherlands, and Switzerland). Also, although there was an overall higher risk among women for worsening of symptoms compared with men, no sex differences were found in Northern European countries, whereas women were at increased risk of worsening in frailty state compared with men in Southern European countries and in Belgium. A systematic review of three studies concluded that studies on frailty trajectories are rare and the results, as for prevalence and incidence rates, highly heterogeneous and dependent on the population and the setting (O'Caoimh et al. 2018).

3.6 Conclusion

In summary, frailty is widely spread in the elderly population worldwide. Depending on the instrument that was used to determine frailty, the calculated prevalence will vary. Studies have shown that prevalence rates are more comparable when the physical frailty index as defined by Fried and colleagues is used than a broader definition that also covers social and psychosocial aspects. However, not only the instrument used, but also geographic variation has been observed independent of the assessment instrument. Prevalence rates in the community-dwelling population tend to be higher in lower-income countries compared with higher-income countries and one of the underlying reasons might be that in lower-income countries fewer older, and potentially frail, people live in nurseries than in higher-income countries. Contributing to differences between studies are different proportions of men and women and different age distributions. Other factors, such as nutritional status, depression, but also ethnic background, are important. Few studies have, however, been conducted on the progression of frailty. Although it has been shown that frailty status of individuals may improve, it is currently unclear who is more likely to improve and why.

References

Avila-Funes JA, Amieva H, Barberger-Gateau P, Le Goff M, Raoux N, Ritchie K et al (2009) Cognitive impairment improves the predictive validity of the phenotype of frailty for adverse health outcomes: the three-city study. J Am Geriatr Soc 57(3):453–461

Buta BJ, Walston JD, Godino JG, Park M, Kalyani RR, Xue QL et al (2016) Frailty assessment instruments: systematic characterization of the uses and contexts of highly-cited instruments. Ageing Res Rev. 26:53–61

Choi J, Ahn A, Kim S, Won CW (2015) Global prevalence of physical frailty by Fried's criteria in community-dwelling elderly with national population-based surveys. J Am Med Dir Assoc 16 (7):548–550

Clegg A, Young J, Iliffe S, Rikkert MO, Rockwood K (2013) Frailty in elderly people. Lancet 381 (9868):752–762

Collard RM, Boter H, Schoevers RA, Oude Voshaar RC (2012) Prevalence of frailty in community-dwelling older persons: a systematic review. J Am Geriatr Soc 60(8):1487–1492

Collerton J, Martin-Ruiz C, Davies K, Hilkens CM, Isaacs J, Kolenda C et al (2012) Frailty and the role of inflammation, immunosenescence and cellular ageing in the very old: cross-sectional findings from the Newcastle 85 + Study. Mech Ageing Dev 133 (6):456–466

Etman A, Burdorf A, Van der Cammen TJ, Mackenbach JP, Van Lenthe FJ (2012) Socio-demographic determinants of worsening in frailty among community-dwelling older people in 11 European countries. J Epidemiol Commun Health 66(12): 1116–1121

Feng Z, Lugtenberg M, Franse C, Fang X, Hu S, Jin C et al (2017) Risk factors and protective factors associated with incident or increase of frailty among community-dwelling older adults: a systematic review of longitudinal studies. PLoS ONE 12(6):e0178383

Fried LP, Tangen CM, Walston J, Newman AB, Hirsch C, Gottdiener J et al (2001) Frailty in older adults: evidence for a phenotype. J Gerontol A Biol Sci Med Sci 56(3):M146–M156

Galluzzo L, O'Caoimh R, Rodriguez-Laso A, Beltzer N, Ranhoff AH, Van der Heyden J et al (2018) Incidence of frailty: a systematic review of scientific literature from a public health perspective. Ann Ist Super Sanita 54(3):239–245

Hirsch C, Anderson ML, Newman A, Kop W, Jackson S, Gottdiener J et al (2006) The association of race with frailty: the cardiovascular health study. Ann Epidemiol 16(7):545–553

Hyde Z, Flicker L, Smith K, Atkinson D, Fenner S, Skeaf L et al (2016) Prevalence and incidence of frailty in Aboriginal Australians, and associations with mortality and disability. Maturitas 87:89–94

Jurschik P, Nunin C, Botigue T, Escobar MA, Lavedan A, Viladrosa M (2012) Prevalence of frailty and factors associated with frailty in the elderly population of Lleida, Spain: the FRALLE survey. Arch Gerontol Geriatr 55(3):625–631

Li G, Thabane L, Papaioannou A, Ioannidis G, Levine MA, Adachi JD (2017) An overview of osteoporosis and frailty in the elderly. BMC Musculoskelet Disord 18(1):46

Mitnitski AB, Graham JE, Mogilner AJ, Rockwood K (2002) Frailty, fitness and late-life mortality in relation to chronological and biological age. BMC Geriatr 2:1

Nguyen TN, Cumming RG, Hilmer SN (2015) A review of frailty in developing countries. J Nutr Health Aging. 19(9):941–946

O'Caoimh R, Galluzzo L, Rodriguez-Laso A, Van der Heyden J, Ranhoff AH, Carcaillon-Bentata L et al (2018) Transitions and trajectories in frailty states over time: a systematic review of the European Joint Action ADVANTAGE. Ann Ist Super Sanita 54 (3):246–252

Ottenbacher KJ, Ostir GV, Peek MK, Snih SA, Raji MA, Markides KS (2005) Frailty in older Mexican Americans. J Am Geriatr Soc 53(9):1524–1531

Pena FG, Theou O, Wallace L, Brothers TD, Gill TM, Gahbauer EA et al (2014) Comparison of alternate scoring of variables on the performance of the frailty index. BMC Geriatr 14:25

Romero-Ortuno R (2013) The SHARE operationalized frailty phenotype: a comparison of two approaches. Eur Geriatr Med 4(4)

Rothman MD, Leo-Summers L, Gill TM (2008) Prognostic significance of potential frailty criteria. J Am Geriatr Soc 56(12):2211–2216

Santos-Eggimann B, Cuenoud P, Spagnoli J, Junod J (2009) Prevalence of frailty in middle-aged and older community-dwelling Europeans living in 10 countries. J Gerontol A Biol Sci Med Sci 64(6):675–681

Shivappa N, Stubbs B, Hebert JR, Cesari M, Schofield P, Soysal P et al (2018) The relationship between the dietary inflammatory index and incident frailty: a longitudinal cohort study. J Am Med Dir Assoc 19 (1):77–82

Siriwardhana DD, Hardoon S, Rait G, Weerasinghe MC, Walters KR (2018) Prevalence of frailty and prefrailty among community-dwelling older adults in low-income and middle-income countries: a systematic review and meta-analysis. BMJ Open 8(3): e018195

Theou O, Brothers TD, Rockwood MR, Haardt D, Mitnitski A, Rockwood K (2013) Exploring the relationship between national economic indicators and relative fitness and frailty in middle-aged and older Europeans. Age Ageing 42(5):614–619

Trevisan C, Veronese N, Maggi S, Baggio G, De Rui M, Bolzetta F et al (2016) Marital status and frailty in older people: gender differences in the progetto veneto anziani longitudinal study. J Womens Health (Larchmt) 25(6):630–637

Verlaan S, Ligthart-Melis GC, Wijers SLJ, Cederholm T, Maier AB, de van der Schueren MAE (2017) High prevalence of physical frailty among community-dwelling malnourished older adults-A systematic review and meta-analysis. J Am Med Dir Assoc 18(5):374–382

Wu C, Kim DH, Xue QL, Lee DSH, Varadhan R, Odden MC (2018) Association of frailty with recovery from disability among community-dwelling older adults: results from two large U.S. cohorts. J Gerontol A Biol Sci Med Sci 74(4):575–581

4 Epidemiology of Cardiovascular Diseases in the Elderly

Marianna Noale, Federica Limongi and Stefania Maggi

Abstract

This chapter focuses on the epidemiology of cardiovascular diseases in elderly adults who are 65 or older. Risk factors for morbidity and mortality, as well as variables associated with disability and physical and social functional decline in the elderly individuals are considered. Modifiable risk factors, such as life habits are differentiated from unmodifiable ones, such as age and sex. The chapter concentrates in particular on the impact of hypertension, dyslipidemia and diabetes on cardiovascular diseases and mortality, as well as the effect of cigarettes smoking, physical activity, obesity and isolation on cardiovascular diseases and quality of life. The results demonstrate that cardiovascular diseases are not necessarily a consequence of aging; instead, they are often linked to modifiable risk factors. We can conclude that specific, targeted prevention interventions should preferably be implemented when individuals are young, but they are also useful in the elderly not only to prolong life but also to improve their quality of life.

Keywords

Cardiovascular diseases · Epidemiology · Elderly adults

4.1 Introduction

This chapter focuses on risk factors for morbidity, disability and mortality in elderly adults, who are defined here as individuals who are 65 and older. Risk factors are usually defined as the variables whose presence in an individual or in a population raises the probability of death or of developing a morbid condition with respect to that in a risk-free individual/population. Geriatricians are generally interested in investigating not only risk factors for death or disease but also variables that predict disability and physical, psychiatric and social functional decline in elderly subjects. Thus, alongside classic factors such as high blood pressure and malnutrition, they are also concerned with variables that are specific to elderly persons such as loneliness and social isolation (Valtorta et al. 2018).

Risk factors are generally classified as modifiable (life habits, environmental, etc.) or unmodifiable (age, sex, familiarity). Modifiable factors are considered critical as far as prevention is concerned because specific, targeted interventions may be able to attenuate the burden of risk.

M. Noale (✉) · F. Limongi · S. Maggi
National Research Council (CNR), Neuroscience Institute, Aging Branch, Padua, Italy
e-mail: marianna.noale@in.cnr.it

N. Veronese (ed.), *Frailty and Cardiovascular Diseases*, Advances in Experimental Medicine and Biology 1216, https://doi.org/10.1007/978-3-030-33330-0_4

Skepticism about the utility of efforts made to modify traditional cardiovascular risk factors such as smoking, high blood pressure and hypercholesterolemia in elderly adults has long existed. Some doubts are based upon the conviction that it is impossible to change deeply rooted habits and that hypertension and dyslipidemia are normal companions of old age (Pinto 2007; Streja and Streja 2017). There is, instead, a large body of evidence demonstrating that elderly individuals are often receptive to prevention programs aiming to lower their morbidity and mortality for some diseases (Morley and Flaherty 2002). Although risk factors should preferably be corrected or eliminated when subjects are young or middle aged, some data indicate that even elderly individuals can successfully modify some risk factors.

The two categories of cardiovascular risk factors that are considered in this chapter are:

(1) Risk factors for the most frequent causes of disability and of death in elderly adults, such as coronary artery and cardiovascular diseases;
(2) Risk factors for conditions such as iatrogenic illnesses, poverty or isolation that can affect an elderly person's quality of life.

4.2 Cardiovascular Disease

One of the most frequent causes leading to the hospitalization and at times to the death of elderly adults is ischemic heart disease. Figure 4.1 illustrates mortality rates of some age groups of the Italian population. As can be seen, mortality rates are higher in males compared to females, but there is a net increase in the rates of both sexes for the oldest age groups (Health for All (HFA) 2017). Coronary artery disease should not, however, be considered an inevitable consequence of aging. Autopsy reports on even very elderly subjects frequently, in fact, contain descriptions of normal heart valves and heart dimensions and coronary arteries without arterial plaque buildup. As shown in Table 4.1, over the past 25 years ischemic heart disease death rates in Italy have fallen by 26% in males over 75 and by

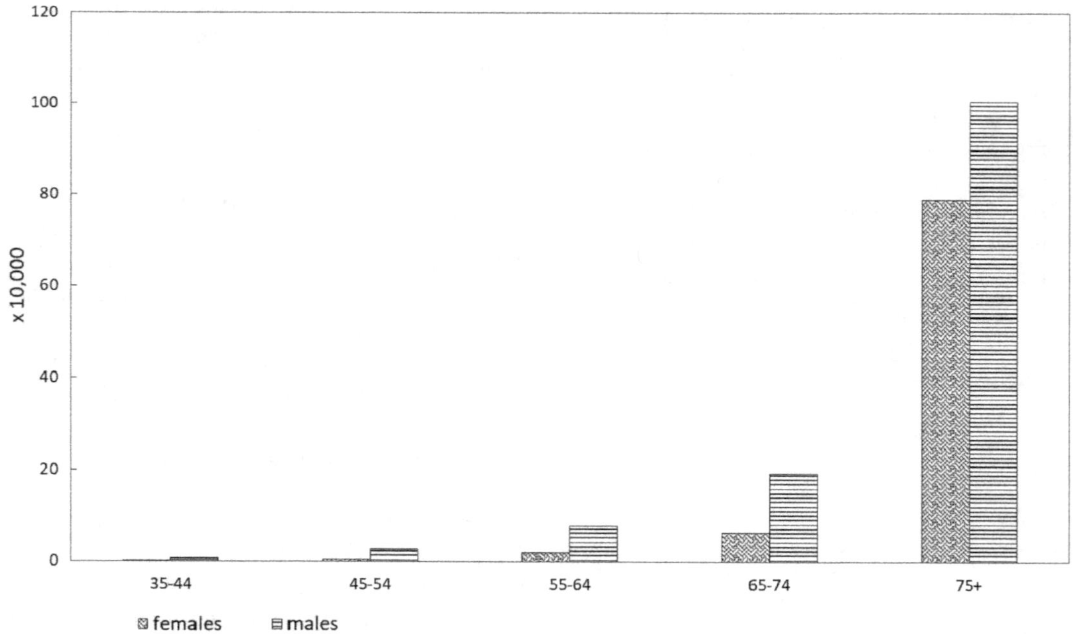

Fig. 4.1 Age-standardized death rates for ischemic heart disease in Italy, 2015

Table 4.1 Standardized mortality rates of ischemic heart disease in Italy between 1990 and 2015

Period	Standardized mortality rates (×10,000)							
	45–54 years	55–64	65–74	75+	45–54 years	55–64	65–74	75+
	Males				Females			
1990	6.80	21.77	51.67	136.19	1.11	5.03	19.75	99.89
1991	7.14	21.53	52.46	142.02	1.16	4.78	18.71	102.95
1992	7.00	19.96	49.86	137.84	1.07	4.46	18.25	101.52
1993	6.50	19.26	50.80	142.57	1.02	4.23	18.46	106.47
1994	6.25	18.47	49.52	144.75	1.03	4.17	18.88	107.37
1995	5.65	17.33	49.17	149.16	1.00	4.09	18.15	110.44
1996	5.47	16.44	47.14	145.27	0.96	3.66	17.25	107.36
1997	5.51	15.61	44.78	141.74	0.97	3.44	16.47	106.71
1998	5.52	15.55	44.53	142.79	0.85	3.68	15.87	107.82
1999	4.73	14.70	40.70	135.86	0.82	3.22	14.98	102.98
2000	4.91	13.35	37.38	130.86	0.75	3.15	13.76	99.31
2001	4.51	12.44	35.45	129.33	0.78	2.93	12.98	95.48
2002	4.43	12.16	35.03	132.41	0.77	2.83	12.34	97.94
2003	4.24	12.37	34.02	139.41	0.68	2.78	12.56	108.95
2004	4.02	11.03	31.08	127.69	0.74	2.50	11.06	95.96
2005	3.80	10.79	29.90	130.08	0.64	2.45	10.73	99.64
2006	3.60	10.06	26.80	120.22	0.61	2.41	9.54	92.33
2007	3.41	9.40	25.18	119.10	0.64	2.24	9.16	92.56
2008	3.31	9.81	24.40	118.08	0.62	2.09	8.34	91.48
2009	3.09	9.12	22.89	114.53	0.55	2.14	8.25	87.52
2010	3.08	8.81	22.46	110.43	0.59	1.86	7.44	83.94
2011	2.86	9.04	22.16	111.24	0.57	1.99	7.49	87.33
2012	2.69	8.49	21.55	111.94	0.50	2.10	7.22	87.02
2013	2.70	8.00	20.18	104.52	0.49	1.71	6.94	79.65
2014	2.45	7.26	18.95	99.05	0.56	1.77	6.35	75.68
2015	2.66	7.79	19.30	100.40	0.44	1.80	6.22	78.96

Source the December 2017 version of the HFA Database, https://www.istat.it/it/archivio/14562

60% in males between 45 and 74 (Health for All (HFA) 2017). The marked reduction in mortality rates found in the elderly segment of the population confirms that the disease is at least in part preventable.

4.2.1 Hypertension

Although it is commonly thought that blood pressure invariably rises with age, high blood pressure is neither inevitable nor innocuous in elderly persons. Increases in blood pressure in elderly adults are for the most part caused by arterial wall stiffness that naturally occurs as individuals age. Historically, while this pattern was often found in individuals living in industrialized countries, it was a less frequent finding in some primitive, isolated populations (Maddocks 1976) and longitudinal studies did not uncover any increase in the systolic/diastolic pressure in a community of healthy, non-institutionalized elderly persons. High blood pressure is not a normal phenomenon linked to aging (Mueller et al. 2018); it represents instead a pathological process that can be prevented and treated in the elderly person just as in the rest of the population.

The prevalence of high blood pressure (defined as systolic blood pressure values >140 mmHg and diastolic >90 mmHg) is frequently quite elevated in high-income countries, ranging between 41 and 77.5% in persons over 60 with respect to 4.3 and 19.7% in persons younger than 30 (Mills et al. 2016).

The Framingham Study (Franklin and Wong 2013) reported that individuals over 65 whose systolic pressure was over 180 mmHg had a 4–5 times greater risk of coronary artery disease with respect to those whose blood pressure was lower than 120 mmHg. Individuals whose diastolic blood pressure was higher than 105 mmHg presented a mortality risk that was 3–4 times higher with respect to that in individuals with values inferior to 75 mmHg. The study also showed that the risk of coronary artery disease was twice as high in elderly adults with high blood pressure with respect to younger adults with high blood pressure, both for males and females. It has also been demonstrated that elderly patients with hypertension have a higher prevalence of myocardial infarction with respect to their normal-blood-pressure counterparts (Lloyd-Jones et al. 2009).

Treatments with antihypertensive medication significantly reduce stroke, cardiovascular events, and mortality in older adults (Beckett et al. 2011). In particular, the Hypertension in the Very Elderly Trial (HYVET) (Warwick et al. 2015) demonstrated that the antihypertensive treatment could be beneficial also when started after 80 years of age. Findings from the SPRINT trial, moreover, demonstrated that lowering standard blood pressure (SBP) to <130 mmHg in adults 75 or older with high CV risk led to lower rates of fatal and nonfatal major cardiovascular events and all-cause mortality (Wright et al. 2015).

4.2.2 Lipids and Lipoproteins

The concentration of plasma cholesterol increases with age from puberty until 45 to 55 years of age in men and tend to stabilize when they are in their 60 s. In women, cholesterol increases until ten years later and stabilization takes place in women who are in their 70 s. The low-density lipoproteins (LDL), considered the atherogenic lipoproteins, tend, in particular, to diminish after 70 (Félix-Redondo et al. 2013). The decline can be due to a decrease in LDL synthesis due to decreased liver function, but also to a selective survival in older adults with lower levels. HDL, which is considered the protective component, fluctuate less than LDL, especially in men (Félix-Redondo et al. 2013).

It has been hypothesized that a lower prevalence of dyslipidemia in very elderly adults could be due to a variety of factors, such as (Lind et al. 2018):

(1) the selective survival of individuals with normal blood values. According to this theory, those persons with hyperlipidemia died at an earlier age, and this would explain the low prevalence of dyslipidemia in the elderly group.
(2) a cohort effect: persons born at an earlier date could have been exposed to fewer risk factors such as diets containing large quantities of saturated fats with respect to individuals born at a later date.
(3) the awareness to decrease fat intake in the population in more recent years.

According to a review by Félix-Redondo et al. (2013), the prevalence of hypercholesterolemia in elderly adults, considering a cut-off of 240 mg/dl for total cholesterol, ranged from 10% in Thailand to more than 50% in England, and was generally higher in Western countries.

Several studies have reported that hypercholesterolemia continues to be a cardiovascular risk factor even in individuals over 65 (Shanmugasundaram et al. 2010). A meta-analysis published in 2004 uncovered a positive association between hypercholesterolemia and CHD morbidity and mortality in men, but not in women, over 65 years, while for persons aged 80 years or more, an inverse relationship of serum total cholesterol with all-cause mortality was observed (Anum and Adera 2004). The Rotterdam Study found that higher total cholesterol was associated with lower mortality for non-cardiovascular causes in older adults aged 65 years or more, with an inverse association increasing with the increase in age (Newson et al. 2011).

While the association of LDL cholesterol and cardiovascular morbidity and mortality seems to be attenuated at older age, a strong association of HDL cholesterol and outcomes was observed at older age (Odden et al. 2014). In the Uppsala Longitudinal Study of Adult Men (ULSAM), during a follow-up of 40 years LDL cholesterol remained a strong risk factor for myocardial infarction, and became significant at older ages also for ischemic stroke; HDL-cholesterol seemed to be protective mainly at middle ages (Lind et al. 2018).

Current recommendations from the National Cholesterol Education Program Adult Treatment Panel (NCEP ATP-III) are for treatment of LDL cholesterol to values <100 mg/dl for patients with known CHD or CHD risk equivalents such as diabetes mellitus (Expert Panel 2001). Considering that the causes of dyslipidemia may be linked to lifestyles, placing patients on an appropriate diet should be considered the first step in preventing and treating hypercholesterolemia (Félix-Redondo et al. 2013).

4.2.3 Diabetes

Type 2 Diabetes is a risk factor for cardiovascular morbidity and mortality in the elderly population. Even though the association between coronary disease and diabetes is not as strong in older with respect to younger populations, it is an important risk factor for congestive heart failure, especially in women, as well as for peripheral arterial disease and claudication (Dhingra and Vasan 2011; Rhee and Kim 2015). The mortality for cardiovascular morbidity is four times higher in diabetic than in non-diabetic women (Collins et al. 2016). Contributors to cardiovascular risk in diabetes include hyperglycemia, dyslipidemia, obesity, insulin resistance, inflammation and hypertension (Halter et al. 2014).

There is however little evidence that lowering blood glucose levels by prescribing insulin or oral anti-diabetic drugs affects the development of cardiovascular complications or mortality. But given the high prevalence of risk factors associated to diabetes, it seems essential in any case to monitor blood glucose levels and to treat concomitant risk factors (Yakaryilmaz and Öztürk 2017).

4.2.4 Cigarette Smoking

The causal relationship between smoking and cardiovascular morbidity and mortality has been amply investigated and confirmed in young adults, but despite being a relevant modifiable risk factor, few prospective studies investigated the effect of cigarettes smoking on cardiovascular outcomes at advanced age (Gellert et al. 2013). These studies suggest that even in later life, smoking is a risk factor for cardiovascular deaths and disease, and that smoking cessation could still be beneficial.

The influence of cigarette smoking on cardiovascular morbidity is mediated by different pathophysiological pathways, including vasomotor dysfunction, inflammation, and smooth muscle proliferation (Ambrose and Barua 2004).

A meta-analysis by Mons et al. (2015) considering persons aged 60 years and older, evidenced that cigarettes smoking was strongly associated with acute coronary events, stroke, and cardiovascular deaths. The hazard of cardiovascular mortality was double among smokers with respect to never smokers, with an excess risk increasing with higher levels of cigarette consumption. These data confirm that it is important to convince elderly smokers to give up smoking and that it is possible to change habits even at an elderly age.

4.2.5 Physical Activity

The idea that physical activity has beneficial effects on several health conditions (cardiovascular pathology, osteoporosis and obesity, etc.) has been widely accepted, and a decline in physical activity has been demonstrated to lead to increased risk of cardiovascular, cerebrovascular and coronary heart diseases (Iijima et al. 2012). Unfortunately, recent reports dealt with middle-aged populations and little is known about the correlation between physical activity and cardiovascular events in elderly persons.

The positive effect of physical activity on cardiovascular disease could be attributed to a direct action on the cardiovascular system or to an indirect one on specific risk factors. It has already been established, for example, that physical activity is inversely associated to blood cholesterol levels and to blood pressure values in the elderly and it is directly associated to glucose tolerance, to insulin resistance, and to neuropsychological performance. It has also been reported that physical activity has a positive effect on pulmonary ventilation and oxygenation (Fiogbé et al. 2017).

4.2.6 Obesity

Most agree that there is a positive association between overweight/obesity and cardiovascular risk in young adults (Ebbert et al. 2014). But an association between these factors in elderly adults continues to be a controversial issue (Maggi et al. 2015). According to data from the Framingham study, the cardiovascular mortality risk was higher in both the overweight and obese individuals in both sexes. The mortality of individuals with a high body mass index (BMI) (above the 70th percentile) was found to be 100% higher in the women and 40% higher in the men with respect to that in individuals whose weight fell between the 30–49th percentile (Long and Fox 2016). Recent studies have shown that the relationship between BMI and cardiovascular morbidity and mortality in elderly subjects can be expressed in the form of a U-shaped curve, suggesting that unilateral interventions in weight reduction in the elderly may be inappropriate (Wu et al. 2014).

Environmental factors are likely to be major contributors to the current obesity epidemic, together with biological predisposition. It is certain that obesity develops when there is a positive imbalance between energy intake and energy expenditure, but the relative contribution of these factors is poorly understood. Evidence supports the contribution of both excess energy intake and decreased energy expenditure in determining obesity. With regard to diet, it has been extensively demonstrated that healthy dietary patterns, such as the Mediterranean diet, have a positive impact not only in preventing obesity at any age, but also preventing CVD in the aged individuals (Boccardi et al. 2018).

4.3 Isolation and Poverty

The lack of social and familial support systems is considered a risk factor for morbidity and mortality for elderly persons. Elderly widows and widowers have, in fact, a higher morbidity and mortality with respect to elderly persons who are living with their husband/wife; this has been explained by the state of isolation in which these individuals find themselves or by the stress that accompanies a period of mourning (Brenn and Ytterstad 2016).

According to the Alameda County Study, elderly individuals with few social contacts are twice as likely to die with respect to those who are still in touch with friends and relatives (Patterson and Veenstra 2010). This association is generally explained by the fact that social ties promote physical activity, improve psychological status, provide an essential support during illness, and all of these help individuals regain their health.

Likewise poverty, in particular changes in an individual's social-economic status (SES), which refers to education, income, occupation, living conditions, income, and other aspects that may be linked to retirement, are associated to higher mortality and morbidity. Several studies have reported an inverse association between SES and CVD mortality, independently from several CVD risk factors and from access to health care. Factors such as stress levels, the presence of negative psychosocial factors and less access to medical care may also explain the relationship between low SES and CVD (Carrino et al. 2018).

Given the importance of socio-economic conditions on the quality of life of all individuals and thus also of elderly adults, they need to be considered when prevention interventions to promote physical and psychological health are being planned.

4.3.1 Cerebrovascular Diseases

Cerebrovascular diseases, which represent the second leading cause of death globally, include ischemic and hemorrhagic stroke and transient ischemic attacks (Tang et al. 2014).

Figure 4.2 shows the standardized mortality rates for cerebrovascular diseases in the Italian population (Health for All (HFA) 2017). Just as for ischemic heart disease, in Italy, mortality is higher in the males with respect to the females with the exception of individuals 75 and over and there is a net increase in mortality as people age. Although the mortality rate has fallen over the last 30 years, strokes are the third cause of death in elderly populations. As can be seen in Table 4.2, there has been a 50% decline in mortality over the last quarter century in males in Italy over 75 and a 69% decline in males falling into the 65–74 age group. There has been a 42% decline in women 75 and over and a 70% decline in the 65–74 age group.

The risk factors are, for the most part, the same as those for cardiovascular disorders, or in other words, hypertension, diabetes, hypercholesterolemia, obesity and smoking (O'Donnell et al. 2016). Some risk factors such as dietary habits, poor physical function, and substance abuse are modifiable (Jauch et al. 2013).

Data from the INTERSTROKE study, demonstrated that ten potentially modifiable risk factors, including hypertension, waist-to-hip ration, diet, physical activity, diabetes and alcohol intake, were associated with 90% of the population attributable risk of acute stroke and intracerebral hemorrhage in each major region of the world, in ethnic groups, in men and women, and in different age group including persons aged 55 years or more (O'Donnell et al. 2016).

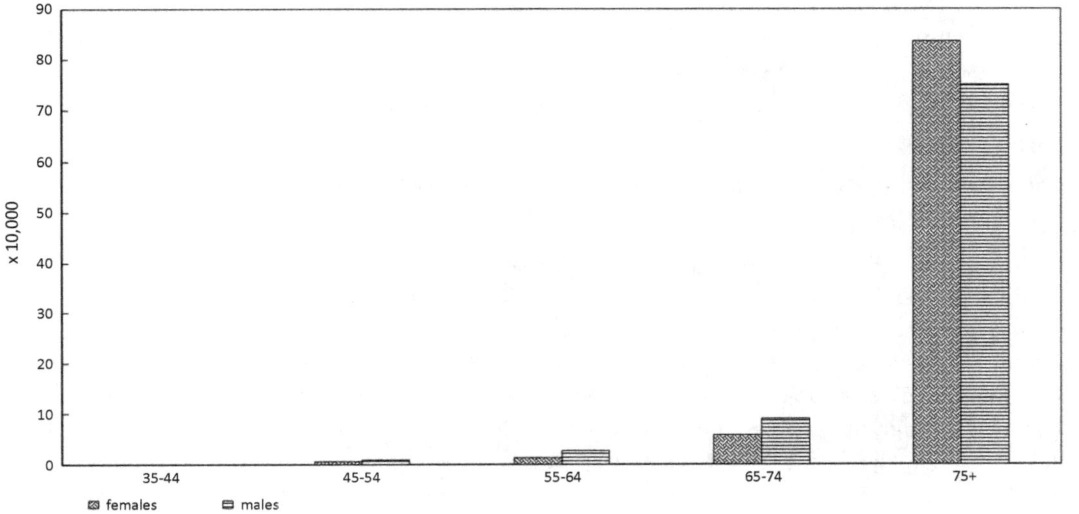

Fig. 4.2 Standardized Mortality rates for cerebrovascular disorders in the Italian population, 2015

Table 4.2 Mortality rates due to cerebrovascular disorders in the Italian population between 1990 and 2015

Period	Standardized mortality rates (×10,000)							
	45–54 years	55–64	65–74	75+	45–54 years	55–64	65–74	75+
	Males				Females			
1990	2.29	8.04	28.90	152.44	1.38	4.38	19.08	145.54
1991	2.24	7.81	27.72	159.70	1.51	4.29	17.69	148.08
1992	2.17	7.63	26.58	151.57	1.30	3.87	17.01	147.37
1993	2.14	6.46	26.01	159.23	1.24	3.83	16.97	151.87
1994	1.81	6.47	25.9	156.39	1.22	3.57	17.03	153.22
1995	1.80	6.01	23.54	144.17	1.19	3.24	15.58	140.33
1996	1.60	5.35	22.78	134.96	1.15	3.2	14.31	132.17
1997	1.61	5.33	22.28	134.29	1.09	2.86	13.90	131.53
1998	1.58	5.32	21.73	133.90	1.17	2.78	13.94	130.52
1999	1.55	4.77	20.39	122.58	0.95	2.62	12.29	122.61
2000	1.51	4.61	19.48	119.92	0.98	2.45	11.63	118.87
2001	1.47	4.45	17.57	113.45	0.99	2.32	10.78	112.81
2002	1.38	4.05	16.71	112.35	0.94	2.40	10.1	110.91
2003	1.33	4.16	16.19	113.14	0.78	2.08	10.12	115.08
2004	1.08	3.40	14.66	95.71	0.79	1.78	8.55	96.82
2005	1.03	3.39	13.65	98.24	0.71	1.79	8.25	99.17
2006	1.05	3.27	12.75	92.11	0.73	1.76	7.77	94.53
2007	1.06	3.02	11.93	90.13	0.60	1.73	7.40	94.76
2008	0.97	3.12	12.18	92.30	0.75	1.60	7.46	95.11
2009	0.94	3.09	11.80	88.47	0.68	1.56	7.10	93.90
2010	0.94	2.78	11.11	83.53	0.63	1.53	6.37	88.52
2011	0.92	2.86	10.35	82.11	0.69	1.63	6.36	87.24
2012	0.83	2.68	10.16	81.28	0.62	1.63	6.36	88.34
2013	0.80	2.53	9.46	75.81	0.57	1.50	5.79	81.62
2014	0.91	2.46	8.87	71.09	0.61	1.53	5.76	77.97
2015	0.88	2.63	9.08	75.03	0.59	1.30	5.78	83.59

Source December 2017 version of the HFA Database, https://www.istat.it/it/archivio/14562

Treating hypertension can undoubtedly be considered an efficacious preventive measure for cerebrovascular disease, and a significant reduction in cerebrovascular disorders has, in fact, been found in elderly subjects who are receiving treatment for high blood pressure (Rubio-Guerra and Duran-Salgado 2015; Castilla-Guerra et al. 2012).

4.4 Conclusion

This chapter presents epidemiological data on some risk factors for morbidity and mortality in the elderly population. Good health status clearly does not depend on biological factors alone but is also linked to socio-economic aspects. The results outlined here are encouraging because they show that morbidity is not necessarily a consequence of aging but is due to specific, often modifiable risk factors.

It seems clear then that primary and secondary prevention interventions should be implemented not only to prolong life but to improve quality of life and to reduce morbidity and physical and social dependence.

References

Ambrose JA, Barua RS (2004) The pathophysiology of cigarette smoking and cardiovascular disease: an update. J Am Coll Cardiol 43:1731–1737

Anum EA, Adera T (2004) Hypercholesterolemia and coronary heart disease in the elderly: a meta-analysis. Ann Epidemiol 14(9):705–721

Beckett N, Peters R, Tuomilehto J, Swift C, Sever P, Potter J et al (2011) Immediate and late benefits of treating very elderly people with hypertension: results from the active treatment extension to Hypertension in the very elderly randomised controlled trial. BMJ 344: d7541

Boccardi V, Calvani R, Limongi F, Marseglia A, Mason A, Noale M, Rogoli D et al (2018) Consensus paper on the "executive summary of the international conference on Mediterranean diet and health: a lifelong approach" an Italian initiative supported by the Mediterranean Diet Foundation and the Menarini Foundation. Nutrition 51–52:38–45

Brenn T, Ytterstad E (2016) Increased risk of death immediately after losing a spouse: cause-specific mortality following widowhood in Norway. Prev Med 89:251–256

Carrino L, Maggi S, Veronese N (2018) Socio-economic issues and CVD. In: ESC textbook of cardiovascular medicine, 3rd edn. Oxford University Press (OUP)

Castilla-Guerra L, Fernández-Moreno Mdel C, Romera-Tellado M, Alvarez-Suero J (2012) Primary stroke prevention in the elderly: current evidence in the treatment of arterial hypertension. Rev Esp Geriatr Gerontol 47:119–124

Collins P, Webb CM, de Villiers TJ, Stevenson JC, Panay N, Baber RJ (2016) Cardiovascular risk assessment in women—an update. Climacteric 19:329–336

Dhingra R, Vasan RS (2011) Diabetes and the risk of heart failure. Heart Fail Clin 8:125–133

Ebbert JO, Elrashidi MY, Jensen MD (2014) Managing overweight and obesity in adults to reduce cardiovascular disease risk. Curr Atheroscler Rep 16:445

Expert Panel on Detection, Evaluation, and Treatment of High Blood Cholesterol in Adults (2001) Executive Summary of the Third Report of The National Cholesterol Education Program (NCEP) Expert Panel on Detection, Evaluation and Treatment of High Blood Cholesterol in Adults (Adult Treatment Panel III). JAMA 285:2486–2497

Félix-Redondo FJ, Grau M, Fernández-Bergés D (2013) Cholesterol and cardiovascular disease in the elderly. Facts and gaps. Aging Dis 4:154–169

Fiogbé E, de Vassimon-Barroso V, de Medeiros Takahashi AC (2017) Exercise training in older adults, what effects on muscle oxygenation. A systematic review. Arch Gerontol Geriatr 71:89–98

Franklin SS, Wong ND (2013) Hypertension and cardiovascular disease: contributions of the Framingham Heart Study. Glob Heart 8:49–57

Gellert C, Schöttker B, Müller H, Holleczek B, Brenner H (2013) Impact of smoking and quitting on cardiovascular outcomes and risk advancement periods among older adults. Eur J Epidemiol 28:649–658

Halter JB, Musi N, McFarland Horne F, Crandall JP, Goldberg A, Harkless L, Hazzard WR et al (2014) Diabetes and cardiovascular disease in older adults: current status and future directions. Diabetes 63:2578–2589

Health for All (HFA) (2017) Database (version of December 2017). https://www.istat.it/it/archivio/14562. Accessed 09 Nov 2018

Iijima K, Iimuro S, Shinozaki T, Ohashi Y, Sakurai T, Umegaki H, Araki A et al (2012) Lower physical activity is a strong predictor of cardiovascular events in elderly patients with type 2 diabetes mellitus beyond traditional risk factors: the Japanese Elderly Diabetes Intervention Trial. Geriatr Gerontol Int 12:77–87

Jauch EC, Saver JL, Adams HP Jr, Bruno A, Connors JJ, Demaerschalk BM et al (2013) Guidelines for the early management of patients with acute ischemic stroke: a guideline for healthcare professionals from the American Heart Association/American Stroke Association. Stroke 44:870–947

Lind L, Sundström J, Ärnlöv J, Lampa E (2018) Impact of aging on the strength of cardiovascular risk factors: a longitudinal study over 40 years. J Am Heart Assoc 7. pii: e007061

Lloyd-Jones D, Adams R, Carnethon M, De Simone G, Ferguson TB, Flegal K et al (2009) Heart disease and stroke statistics–2009 update: a report from the American Heart Association Statistics Committee and Stroke Statistics Subcommittee. Circulation 119: e21–e181

Long MT, Fox CS (2016) The Framingham Heart Study–67 years of discovery in metabolic disease. Nat Rev Endocrinol 12:177–183

Maddocks I (1976) Possible absence of essential hypertension in two complete Pacific Island population. Lancet 2:327

Maggi S, Busetto L, Noale M, Limongi F, Crepaldi G (2015) Obesity: definition and epidemiology. In: Lenzi A (ed) Multidisciplinary approach to obesity: from assessment to treatment. Springer International Publishing Switzerland

Mills KT, Bundy JD, Kelly TN, Reed JE, Kearney PM, Reynolds K et al (2016) Global disparities of hypertension prevalence and control: a systematic analysis of population-based studies from 90 countries. Circulation 134:441–450

Mons U, Müezzinler A, Gellert C, Schöttker B, Abnet CC, Bobak M, de Groot L et al (2015) Impact of smoking and smoking cessation on cardiovascular events and mortality among older adults: meta-analysis of individual participant data from prospective cohort studies of the CHANCES consortium. BMJ 350:h1551

Morley JE, Flaherty JH (2002) It's never too late: health promotion and illness prevention in older persons. J Gerontol A Biol Sci Med Sci 57:M338–M342

Mueller NT, Noya-Alarcon O, Contreras M, Appel LJ, Dominguez-Bello MG (2018) Association of age with blood pressure across the lifespan in isolated Yanomami and Yekwana Villages. JAMA Cardiol. https://doi.org/10.1001/jamacardio.2018.3676

Newson RS, Felix JF, Heeringa J, Hofman A, Witteman JC, Tiemeier H (2011) Association between serum cholesterol and noncardiovascular mortality in older age. J Am Geriatr Soc 59:1779–1785

O'Donnell MJ, Chin SL, Rangarajan S, Xavier D, Liu L, Zhang H et al (2016) Global and regional effects of potentially modifiable risk factors associated with acute stroke in 32 countries (INTERSTROKE): a case-control study. Lancet 388:761–775

Odden MC, Shlipak MG, Whitson HE, Katz R, Kearney PM, defilippi C, Shastri S, Sarnak MJ et al (2014) Risk factors for cardiovascular disease across the spectrum of older age: the Cardiovascular Health Study. Atherosclerosis 237:336–42

Patterson AC, Veenstra G (2010) Loneliness and risk of mortality: a longitudinal investigation in Alameda County, California. Soc Sci Med 71:181–186

Pinto E (2007) Blood pressure and ageing. Postgrad Med J 83:109–114

Rhee SY, Kim YS (2015) Peripheral arterial disease in patients with type 2 diabetes mellitus. Diabetes Metab J 39:283–290

Rubio-Guerra AF, Duran-Salgado MB (2015) Recommendations for the treatment of hypertension in elderly people. Cardiovasc Hematol Agents Med Chem 12:146–151

Shanmugasundaram M, Rough SJ, Alpert JS (2010) Dyslipidemia in the elderly: should it be treated? Clin Cardiol 33:4–9

Streja D, Streja E (2017) Management of dyslipidemia in the elderly. In: De Groot LJ, Chrousos G, Dungan K, Feingold KR, Grossman A, Hershman JM, Koch C et al (eds) Endotext [Internet]. MDText.com, Inc., South Dartmouth (MA), 2000–2017

Tang Z, Zhou T, Luo Y, Xie C, Huo D, Tao L, Pan L et al (2014) Risk factors for cerebrovascular disease mortality among the elderly in Beijing: a competing risk analysis. PLoS ONE 9:e87884

Valtorta NK, Kanaan M, Gilbody S, Hanratty B (2018) Loneliness, social isolation and risk of cardiovascular disease in the English Longitudinal Study of Ageing. Eur J Prev Cardiol 25:1387–1396

Warwick J, Falaschetti E, Rockwood K, Mitnitski A, Thijs L, Beckett N, Bulpitt C, Peters R (2015) No evidence that frailty modifies the positive impact of antihypertensive treatment in very elderly people: an investigation of the impact of frailty upon treatment effect in the Hypertension in the Very Elderly Trial (HYVET) study, a double-blind, placebo-controlled study of antihypertensives in people with hypertension aged 80 and over. BMC Med 13:78

Wright J, Williamson J, Whelton P, Snyder J, Sink K, Rocco M et al (2015) A randomized trial of intensive versus standard blood-pressure control. N Engl J Med 373:2103–2116

Wu CY, Chou YC, Huang N, Chou YJ, Hu HY, Li CP (2014) Association of body mass index with all-cause and cardiovascular disease mortality in the elderly. PLoS ONE 9(7):e102589

Yakaryılmaz FD, Öztürk ZA (2017) Treatment of type 2 diabetes mellitus in the elderly. World J Diabetes 8:278–285

Risk Factors for Frailty and Cardiovascular Diseases: Are They the Same?

5

Karolina Piotrowicz and Jerzy Gąsowski

Abstract

Cardiovascular disease burden increases with the increasing age of populations. Also, with increasing longevity, some individuals are ageing along an unfavourable path developing frailty syndrome. Epidemiologic studies indicate that frailty is overrepresented among the persons with cardiovascular disease. On the other hand, frail subjects tend to be burdened with cardiovascular disease to a greater degree than their biologically better-off peers. Hypertension, diabetes, and obesity, especially abdominal, and at least some other risk factors appear to be shared between frailty and cardiovascular disease. The probable common underlying pathophysiologic feature is inflammation and associated phenomena, possibly having its root in the inflammageing. We discuss these issues based on the results of original studies, comprehensive literature reviews, and metaanalyses, by hundreds of dedicated researchers worldwide.

Keywords

Epidemiology · Risk factors · Frailty · Cardiovascular disease

K. Piotrowicz · J. Gąsowski (✉)
Department of Internal Medicine and Gerontology, Medical College, Jagiellonian University, Kraków, Poland
e-mail: jerzy.gasowski@uj.edu.pl

5.1 Introduction

The burden of cardiovascular disease increases with advancing age. For all entities from hypertension and cardiovascular risk factors to heart failure, cardiovascular events and cardiovascular mortality, the current estimates indicate a steady increase with advancing age (Vasan et al. 2002a, b; GBD 2017 Disease and Injury Incidence and Prevalence Collaborators 2018). At the same time, ageing process is far from being homogenous in all individuals, which bears heavily upon quality of life, morbidity and survival. Poorer physiologic profile, including lower eGFR, low albumin, low sodium, greater white blood cell count, decreased FEV1 has been traced to pre-frailty and frailty phenotypes defined according to Fried criteria (Ramsay et al. 2015). The data from the United States indicate, that while a person at the age of 80 years would on average have eight years to live, the actual survival strongly depends upon the patient's functional status, which in turn is the function of a trajectory of ageing process and the presence of multimorbidity. According to data published by Studenski et al., such 'average' 80 years old male subject walks at a speed of 1.1 m/s. If the walking speed is greater by 0.5 m/s then the prospected survival grows to little under 15 years, whereas it falls to under 5 years when walking speed is 0.2 m/s on average (Studenski et al. 2011). Likewise, the walking speed has been associated in a similarly reverse fashion

N. Veronese (ed.), *Frailty and Cardiovascular Diseases*, Advances in Experimental Medicine and Biology 1216, https://doi.org/10.1007/978-3-030-33330-0_5

with risk of complications of cardiovascular surgery in older persons (Afilalo et al. 2016). This is underpinning the importance of all potential pathologies, acting in a nonspecific way, and their interaction with ageing process to produce functional decline and at the same time to limit survival. The speedier, more aggressive ageing process which induces more pronounced homeostenosis often leads to frailty. The phenotypic feature of frailty and at least some of the cardiovascular disease overlap. Among these, loss of muscle mass and function (sarcopenia), fatigue, or smouldering inflammation come to the fore. Another important, possibly shared, aspect of frailty and cardiovascular disease is cognitive impairment. The question however remains whether the factors implicit in the cardiovascular disease on one hand, and frailty on the other hand overlap. The reports from the INTERHEART and INTERSTROKE studies traced approximately 90% of the variability in cardiovascular risk to 10, classic risk factors (Yusuf et al. 2004; O'Donnell et al. 2010). The American Heart Association launched its Live's Simple 7, aiming at increasing awareness of more appropriate diet ('eat better'), battling against physical inactivity ('get active'), maintaining appropriate weight ('lose weight'), not smoking ('quit smoking'), good metabolic control ('reduce blood sugar', 'control cholesterol'), and having appropriate blood pressure ('manage blood pressure') (American Heart Association 2019). However, whether these factors would equally explain risk of frailty, and in consequence whether battling them will translate into less frailty has not been fully elucidated.

5.2 Frailty and Cardiovascular Disease. A Reciprocal Relation

Numerous studies and several meta-analyses addressed the issue of cardiovascular disease in the context of frailty. Wong et al., in 5,618 participants in the Irish Longitudinal Study on Ageing (TILDA), cross-sectionally addressed the relation between the Systematic Coronary Risk Evaluation (SCORE), Ideal Cardiovascular Health (ICH) , and Cardiovascular Health Metrics (CHM), and the 40-item frailty index. They found a linear relation between SCORE and frailty index. The odds ratio for frailty associated with SCORE indicative of very high risk vs. low-to-moderate was 3.18. Likewise, the poor health indicator vs. good health, based on ICH, had odds ratio for frailty of 3.45 (Wong et al. 2018). Veronese et al. combined data from 10 cross-sectional studies. He found that both pre-frailty and frailty was associated with higher odds ratios for the concomitant cardiovascular disease. The analysis of six longitudinal studies demonstrated that pre-frailty was associated with 23% greater risk of CVD, whereas frailty was associated with 70% greater risk of CVD. Concordant results were obtained for mortality (Veronese et al. 2017a, b). This analysis expanded earlier data from the same group, which indicated that prefrailty defined as fulfilment of up-to two out of five modified Fried criteria was associated in a dose-dependent fashion with greater risk (by 25% for 1 criterion and by 79% for 2 criteria) of CVD (Sergi et al. 2015). Discordant results were demonstrated by Aguayo et al. Based on data of 5294 participants in English Longitudinal Study of Ageing (ELSA) , who were followed for 7 years, Aguayo et al. checked the performance of 35 frailty scores in prediction of cardiovascular disease, cancer and total mortality. The Authors assessed the relative hazard rates of defined outcome measures associated with the frailty scores on a continuous scale. For all outcomes, they found inconsistent results across the scores, with progressive adjustment blunting the statistical significance. The addition of frailty scores on top of age and sex significantly improved the c statistic for all-cause mortality by 0.6–3.1%, however, there was no improvement for the prediction of cardiovascular disease (the age-and-sex-based score C-statistic 0.70) or cancer events (the age-and-sex-based score C-statistic 0.60). This work raises important question as to the practical validity of frailty indexes used in that study in recognizing patients at a greater risk of adverse cardiovascular outcome. Of note the analysis included all major and clinically used indices including the Fried, Rockwood, SPPB, and the 40-item frailty score (Aguayo et al. 2018).

5.3 Cardiovascular Risk Factors and Risk of Frailty

The report from the UK Biobank study (n = 421,000), showed an incremental, dose-dependent relationship between Cardiovascular Risk Score and the increase in risk of frailty as assessed based on Rockwood visual or Fried phenotypic scales (Atkins et al. 2019).

5.3.1 Hypertension

Hypertension is the most important modifiable risk factor of cardiovascular disease. The prevalence of hypertension increases sharply with age, to the effect that the remaining lifetime risk of becoming hypertensive after reaching the age of 55 years is 90% (Vasan et al. 2002a, b; Messerli et al. 2007). Isolated systolic hypertension is the most prevalent form of primary hypertension in the elderly and is associated with higher morbidity and mortality, which is in part associated with higher pulse pressure (Staessen et al. 2000; Gasowski et al. 2002), and Pulse Wave Velocity (PWV) (Zhong et al. 2018). The cross-sectional analysis of data from Framingham Heart Study indicated that PWV increases from robust to pre-frail to frail older persons, which may help linking frailty with increased cardiovascular risk (Orkaby et al. 2019). In the past, it was found that higher levels of blood pressure in midlife translate to greater risk of developing cognitive impairment (Launer et al. 1995). Although, individuals with clinically overt dementia often tend to have lower blood pressures when compared to people free from dementia, when traced back in time, their blood pressures tend to be significantly higher (Skoog et al. 1996). This clinical observation was paralleled by the magnetic resonance data concerning white matter lesions (Korf et al. 2004). Previously we found that subclinical changes in mood and cognition are associated with poorer blood pressure control in a nationwide cohort of older, ambulatory hypertensives (Piotrowicz et al. 2016). Depression and other psychosocial factors have been established as cardiovascular risk factors (Yusuf et al. 2004; O'Donnell et al. 2010). Likewise, the older patients with Post Traumatic Stress Disorder (PTSD) as a result deportations to Siberia during WW2 have been traced to higher cardiovascular risk estimated by greater Pulse Wave Velocity (Walczewska et al. 2011). In a similar group of patients with PTSD, who had high prevalence of depression (73.5%), the prevalence of frailty was also high and amounted 39.7%, and 42% had coronary artery disease. In the same cohort the prevalence of multimorbidity was 91.3% (Piotrowicz et al. 2018). Overall, the prevalence of hypertension in frail persons has recently been estimated in a large meta-analysis by Vetrano et al., at 72%, and the prevalence of frailty among hypertensive patients at 14% (Vetrano et al. 2018). On the other hand, putting the categorical diagnosis of hypertension aside, most data tend to indicate that frail people with advanced age tend to have significantly lower values of blood pressure (Ravindrarajah et al. 2017; Basile et al. 2017), which is in line with the data for association between blood pressure and cognition, and may indicate that hypertension may play a role at earlier stages, before the path of ageing differentiates between frail and robust. Indeed, when developed, frailty tends to have more weight on poor survival, than hypertension per se. In short, a 70-year-old frail male individual has 0.1–1.8 years to live, and female individual of similar age 0.4–5.5 years (Romero-Ortuno et al. 2014). An observation by Gijón-Conde et al. makes it possible to unify low blood pressure, frailty and increased mortality. In a cross-sectional analysis of 1047 Spanish subjects >60 years of age, she found frailty (6%) and disability (8.1%) to be associated with respectively 3.5 and 2.5 mmHg lower daytime, 3.6 and 2.7 mmHg higher night-time SBP, resulting in 3.3 and 2.5% less night-time dipping of SBP, respectively (all $p < 0.02$) (Romero-Ortuno et al. 2014).

5.3.2 Measures of Adiposity

The relation between various measures of adipose tissue and cardiovascular disease has been well documented (Lahey and Khan 2018). From Body Mass Index (BMI) (Lavie et al. 2009), through measures of central obesity (Pischon et al. 2008), through changes in BMI (Bangalore et al. 2017). De Stefani et al., performed a meta-analysis of 5 studies which in total included 178,644 persons. The authors analysed the role of unintentional weight loss in the development of combined cardiovascular events (MACE) or death. In general, the unintentional weight vs. stable weight increased mortality by 38% and non-significantly tended to incidence MACE by 17%. The effect was more pronounced in older persons (81% greater risk of death with weight loss) and persons with comorbidity (38% greater risk upon weight loss) (Bangalore et al. 2017). Of note, and in line with finding by Bangalore et al. (Bangalore et al. 2017), the higher mortality associated with unintentional weight loss was also observed in overweight/obese patients (11% greater risk of mortality with weight loss) (De Stefani et al. 2018). This is despite of the fact that some, mainly cross-sectional analyses find increased BMI to be associated with higher frailty scores (Wong et al. 2018).

The NHANES data for 1999-2004 indicate that the mean (SD) BMI was higher in frail (30.7 (0.49) kg/m^2), as compared to pre-frail (28.3 (0.18) kg/m^2) and robust (27.8 (0.12) kg/m^2). Similar trend was observed for waist circumference from 99.5 cm in robust to 104.7 cm in frail ($p < 0.001$). The total body fat was following the BMI and waist circumference, resulting in frail persons having total body fat of 40.0% compared to 38.3% in pre-frail and 35.9 in robust individuals ($p < 0.001$), indicating potential input of obese sarcopenia in this representative sample of US subjects (Crow et al. 2019). These results are in line with earlier reports mainly from European studies. In a study based on data of over 1.4 million individuals, a U-shaped relationship was found between total mortality and BMI, irrespective of age. Of note, the nadir of the relationship was between the BMI of 18.5 and 24.9 km/m^2 for the group aged 20–49 years, 20.0 and 24.0 km/m^2 for those aged 50–59 years, 20.0–27.4 km/m^2 for the groups aged 60–79 and 80–84 years (Berrington de Gonzalez et al. 2010). Hubbard et al. based on ELSA cohort of 3,055 individuals aged 65 years or more demonstrated similar, U-shaped relation between BMI and frailty, defined according to Fried and Rockwood criteria. Using both criteria for frailty syndrome, lowest prevalence of frailty was found for BMI between 25 and 29.9 kg/m^2 (Hubbard et al. 2010). Indeed, metabolic syndrome and higher levels of leptin are associated with higher prevalence of frailty (Hubbard et al. 2010; Lana et al. 2017).

5.3.3 Smoking

Non-smoking has recently been associated with close to 30% better physical performance in 7,746 with mean age of 55.5 (14.9) years (Landi et al. 2018). In several analyses smoking was cross-sectionally associated with pre-frailty and frailty. The report from the UK Biobank study, performed in individuals aged 37–73 years showed that past smoking was associated with 5% greater risk of pre-frailty and 7% greater risk of frailty. Current smoking was associated with 42% greater risk of pre-frailty and 247% greater risk of frailty (Hanlon et al. 2018). In a cohort of older British men aged 79–92 years, smoking was associated with 17.6% greater risk of pre-frailty and 54% greater risk of frailty (Hanlon et al. 2018). On the other hand, neither the Age, Gene/Environment Susceptibility (AGES) Reykjavik Study with a median follow up of 8.7 years where 3,818 persons aged over 65 years (Veronese et al. 2017a, b), nor the English Longitudinal Study of Ageing (ELSA) which followed for four years 1,726 men and women aged between 60 and 90 years (Gale et al. 2014), did not prospectively confirm this relationship.

5.3.4 Dyslipidemia

In a previously mentioned study by Landi et al., total cholesterol below 5.18 mmol/l, is associated with borderline 17% less risk of poor physical performance defined as the ability to perform 5 unsupported chair-stands within 7.75 s for women and 7.43 s for men (Landi et al. 2018). The data for the cross-sectional association between lipid profile constituents and pre-frailty and frailty turn out to be inconsistent. In a baseline data analysis by Veronese et al., HDL concentration was borderline significantly greater in persons with pre-frailty (61.7 mg/dl) versus non-frail individuals (58.1 mg/dl, $p = 0.04$) (Sergi et al. 2015). However, the ELSA study did not report differences in total cholesterol or HDL between frail and non-frail persons (Gale et al. 2014). The data from the British male cohort indicate that pre-frailty and frailty are associated with higher odds of low HDL and high LDL concentration, although the latter association in the entire studied group was not observed in individuals without concomitant cardiovascular disease (Ramsay et al. 2015). In the Reykjavik Study (AGES), HDL and LDL were marginally lower and triglycerides marginally higher in frail versus non-frail persons. Of note, in this study the two groups did not differ in the intake of lipid-lowering medications. Importantly, in this study, a higher percentage of people affected with frailty had metabolic syndrome (37% vs. 28.4%, $p < 0.0001$) (Veronese et al. 2017a, b).

5.3.5 Diabetes

Diabetes is listed by the European Society of Cardiology (ESC) among the 7 current main targets and goals of the CVD prevention (Piepoli et al. 2016). It accounts for 9.9% population attributable risk (PAR) for coronary heart disease in the international, worldwide, case-control INTERHEART Study (52 countries representing all populated continents, 27,098 participants), and respectively for the PAR of 5% for the association of all stroke in the INTERSTROKE Study (22 countries, 3000 participants) (Yusuf et al. 2004; O'Donnell et al. 2010). Following the numbers discussed in the 2018 joint guidelines of the European Association for the Study of Diabetes (EASAD) and the American Diabetes Association (ADA) on management of hyperglycemia in patients with diabetes type 2, more than one third of the US population aged 65 years and more, suffers from mostly type 2 diabetes. Additional 50% meets the laboratory criteria for pre-diabetes (Menke et al. 2015; Davies et al. 2018). The prevalence of diabetes in frail and pre-frail subjects differs significantly (Veronese et al. 2017a), and for the community dwelling frail subjects ranges from 11% in the US (Khan et al. 2013), 15% in France (the Three City Study) (Avila-Funes et al. 2014), 19% in Italy (Sergi et al. 2015) to 26% in the FIBRA Brazil study (Moreira and Lourenço 2013), 27% in the UK (Ramsay et al. 2015), but also in the US (Eichholzer et al. 2012), and 29% in Taiwan (Lin et al. 2015). For in-hospital frail patients with acute coronary syndrome, diabetes was reported in up to 46% of them (Sanchis et al. 2014), but also in 37% of those burdened with atrial fibrillation (Polidoro et al. 2013). However, the presented results are discordant. Indeed, Ramsay and colleagues in the cross-sectional British Regional Heart Study of the representative sample of 1622 older British men showed a high prevalence of diabetes in frail subjects (almost one third of frail cases) but failed to demonstrate the relation between impaired fasting glucose and both frail and pre-frail syndrome in those with and without established cardiovascular disease (Ramsay et al. 2015). Gale and colleagues in the 4-year follow-up of the ELSA Study proved that those who had been diagnosed with diabetes at the time of baseline assessment, developed physical frailty significantly more often (16.6 and 7.2% of frail and pre-frail subjects respectively, who had been suffered from diabetes on baseline when compared to 6% of those with diabetes but any of the components of physical frailty) (Gale et al. 2014). In the report from the UK Biobank data study diabetes was listed among conditions that were associated with frailty, with the odds of 5.0 (Hanlon et al. 2018). Castrejón-Perez et al., reported a cross-sectional association between diabetes mellitus and frailty in 5,379 older adults with mean (SD) age of 70.3 (7.8) years. The odds of frailty associated with diabetes mellitus were 2.31, and results were compatible across subsamples of hospitalised in previous year (OR

2.32), on insulin and oral glucose lowering medications (OR 5.6) and patients with neuropathy (OR 2.02, all $p < 0.001$) (Castrejón-Pérez et al. 2018). These results may raise suspicion that overachievement of therapeutic goal, possibly associated with episodes of hypoglycaemia may play a role in greater odds of concomitant frailty.

5.3.6 Sedentary Behaviour

Sedentary lifestyle is an established risk factor for cardiovascular disease (Piepoli et al. 2016). Analysis of data from ELSA study supply strong evidence in support of the link between lack of physical activity and frailty. Moderate physical activity defined as car washing, dancing, stretching, moderate-pace walking or gardening, especially from the age of 60 onwards, was associated with significantly lower risk of frailty compared with mild activity and sedentary lifestyles (Rogers et al. 2017). This type of activity is probably much safer for most older persons than the vigorous activity. An umbrella review by Jadczak et al., concludes that multicomponent exercises, resistance training, and the aerobic exercises, balance and flexibility exercises, when instituted in pre-frail and frail patients are effective in increasing gait speed, balance, and physical performance in pre-frail and frail subjects (Jadczak et al. 2018). Similar activities are believed to improve cardiovascular prognosis (Kachur et al. 2017).

5.4 Is There a Common Pathophysiology of Frailty and CVD?

The previously discussed results by Veronese et al., shed some light on the possibility of shared pathological background of frailty and clinical CVD (Veronese et al. 2017a, b). Initially, with adjustment for age only, frailty was increasing the risk of clinical CVD in men and women to a similar degree. However, after adjustment for additional risk factors, and further for subclinical CVD (carotid plaque and total coronary calcifications) the relation remained significant in women (RHR 1.51, $p = 0.006$) but not in men (RHR 1.19, $p = 0.44$). This may be due, at least in part, to the fact that male sex is associated with greater risk of CVD. Of note, of the five constituents of frailty according to Fried criteria, only exhaustion was significantly related to new-onset CVD (Veronese et al. 2017a, b). It may reflect the fact that exhaustion is also an important clinical symptom of CVD, especially in the very old people, in whom it may be a masque of the conditions ranging from stable, through acute coronary artery disease, atrial fibrillation and heart failure. This may further point to the possibility that at least some of the frail or pre-frail older persons, especially men, may already be hosting subclinical CVD (Veronese et al. 2017a, b). The earlier analysis by Sergi et al. demonstrated the low energy expenditure, exhaustion and slow gait have been associated with greater risk of developing CVD (Sergi et al. 2015). The observations by Wong et al., that both diabetes mellitus and smoking are associated with the diagnosis of frailty, and that level of SBP and BMI are positively associated with a 40-item frailty score, lend support to the shared pathogenesis hypothesis. Moreover, in that analysis, 16.4% of the total group were frail, which grew to 42.5% in the octogenarian sub-cohort. In the entire group, 10.7% of individuals without CVD and 43.0% individuals with CVD were frail. This underlines the possibility that speedier vascular ageing may contribute both to the development of cardiovascular disease and frailty (Wong et al. 2018). The interesting data on possible modification or acceleration of processes leading to development of cardiovascular disease were presented by Korada et al., who studied a group of 976 (62% HIV positive) male subjects with mean (SD) age of 54 (O'Donnell et al. 2010) years. The prevalence of frailty was 7.4% in HIV negative men and 14.3% in HIV positive ones. In this pre-old age stratum, based on cardiac CT and coronary CT angiography, frailty only when associated with HIV infection was related to presence of subclinical atherosclerosis assessed with calcium score (>0), total plaque score (>0) and mixed plaque score

(>0). This may indicate the possible modifying role of the immune derangement in both frailty and subclinical atherosclerosis (Korada et al. 2017). In the context of the important data published by Korada et al., one of the possible molecular common denominators of frailty, cardiovascular disease, and HIV/AIDS is the overexpression of interleukin 6 (IL-6) (Nordell et al. 2014).

Low grade inflammation has indeed been traced as a factor important in the development of cardiovascular disease (Ridker et al. 2000; Yang et al. 2009). At the same time, frailty has been associated with such factors as elevated c-reactive protein (CRP) and elevation of IL-6. Velissaris et al., comprehensively reviewed available literature concerning association between CRP and frailty (Velissaris et al. 2017). In some studies CRP was associated with pre-frailty and frailty (Soysal et al. 2016; Saum et al. 2015), including broad range of age (Almeida et al. 2012), octogenarians (Giovannini et al. 2011), and nonagenarians (Tiainen et al. 2010), worse cognitive performance and mortality (Puzianowska-Kuźnicka et al. 2016), adverse association with cognitive function in women (Canon and Crimmins 2011), mortality in multimorbid older persons (Nouvenne et al. 2016), mortality in frail older persons (Giovannini et al. 2011), worse physical performance (Yoshida et al. 2010; Cesari et al. 2004). On the other hand, some studies put a question mark over the existence relation between CRP and frailty in younger old persons (Baylis et al. 2013), in nonagenarians (Jylhä et al. 2007), or a weaker association with CRP and frailty in postmenopausal women (Reiner et al. 2009). Likewise, abundant studies point to the association between IL-6 and frailty (Velissaris et al. 2017), and some between frailty between IL-1Ra (Velissaris et al. 2017).

5.5 Inflammageing—Towards Unifying Theory of Ageing, Frailty, Cardiovascular Disease and Other Age-Related Diseases

Ageing is associated with profound changes at the cellular level, which lead to the development and accumulation, in various organs and organ systems of the senescent cells (Ferrucci and Fabbri 2018). Based on a comprehensive review of the available literature, Ferucci and Fabbri identified these changes to include cell-cycle arrest, loss of the proliferation capacity, global cell enlargement, misshaping of the nuclei, chromatin focal persistent DNA damage response, increase of NF-kappa-B signalling, resistance to apoptosis, increase in cyclin dependent kinase inhibitor 2A ($p16^{INK4A}$) which interferes with replication, and increased activity of lysosomal beta-galactosidase activity (Ferrucci and Fabbri 2018). The accumulation of senescent cells, whether the trigger of prolonged inflammation, its result, or both, is associated with increased expression of inframmation-related molecules including IL-1, IL-1 receptor antagonist protein (IL-1RN), IL-6, IL-8, IL-13, IL-18, CRP, IFNalpha, IFNbeta, TGFbeta, TNF, TNF receptor super family 1a and 1b, and serum amyloid A (Ferrucci and Fabbri 2018; Franceschi et al. 2000; Ferrucci et al. 2010). Likewise, the senescent cells expose the so called Senescence Associated Secretory Phenotype (SASP), which includes secretion of interleukins, chemokins, various growth factors and, of note, metaloproteinases including interstitial colagenase (MMP1) or colagenase 3 (MMP13), which may play an important role in atherosclerotic complications (Wang et al. 2011; Ezhov et al. 2019). Genetic studies tend to indicate that some mutations, for instance in genes encoding IL-6, such as 174 G > C, leading to increased release of IL-6 upon stimulation are associated with higher risk of Alzheimer disease, cardiovascular diseases (Hou et al. 2015) or type 2 diabetes mellitus (Testa et al. 2006). Likewise mutations in genes encoding receptor for IL-6, and CRP, have been traced to increased CVD. An interesting observation was that the SNPs associated with ageing and inflammation cosegregate with those associated with cancer, diabetes, and cardiovascular disease (Jeck et al. 2012; Johnson et al. 2015). Of note, the CDKN2A gene ancoding the $p16^{INK4A}$ is close to a SNP associated with poor physical function (rs284712). Also, the role of some miRNAs has been underlined in the context of accelerated ageing, inflammation and mitochondrial dysfunction, and some were described as protective (Ferrucci and Fabbri 2018; Melzer et al. 2007). Prolonged inflammation can also be triggered by some of the cardiovascular risk factors. For instance: cholesterol crystals may induce the NLRP3 inflammasome which via stimulation to produce IL-1beta may induce atherosclerotic complications. However induced, inflammation down-regulates insulin-like growth factor 1 (IGF1) which has been shown to play role in muscular regeneration and is protective against instability of atherosclerotic plaques (Ridker et al. 2000; Higashi et al. 2016). It was also demonstrated, that inflammation, causes insulin resistance via the TNF receptor superfamily member 1A and the Toll-like-receptor induced activation of Janus kinase, which in turn interferes with insulin signalling. Insulin resistance in turn winds-up inflammation via central obesity (adipocytes release the c-c motif chemokine 2 (CCL2)) and via the tissue accumulation of M1 macrophages (Ferrucci and Fabbri 2018). It is important to stress, that the influence of inflammation on frailty and cardiovascular disease tends to produce, among other, signs and symptoms of fatigue, muscular wasting, low strength, which lends support to possibility that both frailty and cardiovascular disease in the elderly share at least some patophysiologic pathways together with risk factors.

5.6 Conclusions

Despite huge research effort thus far, there are still knowledge gaps in need of addressing. Not all known cardiovascular risk-factors have been examined on the account of being risk factors for frailty. Although we know, that the Mediterranean diet (Guasch-Ferré et al. 2017; Veronese et al. 2018) and regular, moderate physical activity (Jadczak et al. 2018; Kachur et al. 2017) are capable to reduce inflammation, frailty and cardiovascular outcome (Estruch et al. 2013), and that statins, especially in persons with higher CRP, reduce CV risk (Yang et al. 2009) (but not so much frailty itself), we still lack convincing evidence supporting the wide-spread use of particular interventions that would at the same time decrease CV risk and improve functionality, and sarcopenia, maybe, with an exception for physical activity and caloric restriction (Ferrucci and Fabbri 2018). Indeed, the current European cardiovascular prevention guidelines adopt more liberal goals to be achieved in conditions such as hypertension, or diabetes mellitus in the frail population, or, as in the case of dyslipidemia, do not mention fraillty at all (Piepoli et al. 2016).

References

Afilalo J, Kim S, O'Brien S, Brennan JM, Edwards FH, Mack MJ et al (2016) Gait speed and operative mortality in older adults following cardiac surgery. JAMA Cardiol. 1(3):314–321

Aguayo GA, Vaillant MT, Donneau AF, Schritz A, Stranges S, Malisoux L et al (2018) Comparative analysis of the association between 35 frailty scores and cardiovascular events, cancer, and total mortality in an elderly general population in England: An observational study. PLoS Med. 15(3):e1002543

Almeida OP, Norman PE, van Bockxmeer FH, Hankey GJ, Flicker L (2012) CRP 1846G > a polymorphism increases risk of frailty. Maturitas 71(3): 261–266

American Heart Association (2019) Life's Simple 7. Available from: http://heartinsight.heart.org/Lifes-Simple-7/. On-line access on 1 April 2019

Atkins JL, Delgado J, Pilling LC, Bowman K, Masoli JAH, Kuchel GA et al (2019) Impact of low cardiovascular risk profiles on geriatric outcomes: evidence from 421,000 participants in two cohorts. J Gerontol A Biol Sci Med Sci 74(3):350–357

Avila-Funes JA, Meillon C, González-Colaço Harmand M, Tzourio C, Dartigues JF, Amieva H (2014) Association between frailty and carotid central structure changes: the three-city study. J Am Geriatr Soc 62 (10):1906–1911

Bangalore S, Fayyad R, Laskey R, DeMicco DA, Messerli FH, Waters DD (2017) Body-weight fluctuations and outcomes in coronary disease. N Engl J Med 376(14):1332–1340

Basile G, Catalano A, Mandraffino G, Maltese G, Alibrandi A, Ciancio G et al (2017) Relationship between blood pressure and frailty in older hypertensive outpatients. Aging Clin Exp Res 29(5):1049–1053

Baylis D, Bartlett DB, Syddall HE, Ntani G, Gale CR, Cooper C et al (2013) Immune-endocrine biomarkers as predictors of frailty and mortality: a 10-year longitudinal study in community-dwelling older people. Age (Dordr) 35(3):963–971

Berrington de Gonzalez A, Hartge P, Cerhan JR, Flint AJ, Hannan L, MacInnis RJ et al (2010) Body-mass index and mortality among 1.46 Million white adults. N Engl J Med 363(23):2211–2219

Canon ME, Crimmins EM (2011) Sex differences in the association between muscle quality, inflammatory markers, and cognitive decline. J Nutr Health Aging 15(8):695–698

Castrejón-Pérez RC, Aguilar-Salinas CA, Gutiérrez-Robledo LM, Cesari M, Pérez-Zepeda MU (2018) Frailty, diabetes, and the convergence of chronic disease in an age-related condition: a population-based nationwide cross-sectional analysis of the Mexican nutrition and health survey. Aging Clin Exp Res 30(8):935–941

Cesari M, Penninx BW, Pahor M, Lauretani F, Corsi AM, Rhys Williams G et al (2004) Inflammatory markers and physical performance in older persons: the InCHIANTI study. J Gerontol A Biol Sci Med Sci 59(3):242–248

Crow RS, Lohman MC, Titus AJ, Cook SB, Bruce ML, Mackenzie TA et al (2019) Association of obesity and frailty in older adults: NHANES 1999–2004. J Nutr Health Aging. 23(2):138–144

Davies MJ, D'Alessio DA, Fradkin J, Kernan WN, Mathieu C, Mingrone G et al (2018) Management of hyperglycemia in type 2 diabetes, 2018. A consensus report by the american diabetes association (ADA) and the european association for the study of diabetes (EASD). Diabetes Care 41(12):2669–2701

De Stefani FDC, Pietraroia PS, Fernandes-Silva MM, Faria-Neto J, Baena CP (2018) Observational evidence for unintentional weight loss in all-cause mortality and major cardiovascular events: a systematic review and meta-analysis. Sci Rep. 8(1):15447

Eichholzer M, Barbir A, Basaria S, Dobs AS, Feinleib M, Guallar E et al (2012) Serum sex steroid hormones and frailty in older American men of the Third National Health and Nutrition Examination Survey (NHANES III). Aging Male 15(4):208–215

Estruch R, Ros E, Salas-Salvadó J, Covas MI, Corella D, Arós F et al (2013) Primary prevention of cardiovascular disease with a Mediterranean diet. N Engl J Med 368(14):1279–1290

Ezhov M, Safarova M, Afanasieva O, Mitroshkin M, Matchin Y, Pokrovsky S (2019) Matrix metalloproteinase 9 as a predictor of coronary atherosclerotic plaque instability in stable coronary heart disease patients with elevated lipoprotein(a) levels. Biomolecules 9(4):E129

Ferrucci L, Fabbri E (2018) Inflammageing: chronic inflammation in ageing, cardiovascular disease, and frailty. Nat Rev Cardiol 15(9):505–522

Ferrucci L, Semba RD, Guralnik JM, Ershler WB, Bandinelli S, Patel KV et al (2010) Proinflammatory state, hepcidin, and anemia in older persons. Blood 115(18):3810–3816

Franceschi C, Bonafè M, Valensin S, Olivieri F, De Luca M, Ottaviani E et al (2000) Inflammaging. An evolutionary perspective on immunosenescence. Ann N Y Acad Sci 908:244–254

Gale CR, Cooper C, Sayer AA (2014) Framingham cardiovascular disease risk scores and incident frailty: the English longitudinal study of ageing. Age (Dordr) 36(4):9692

Gasowski J, Fagard RH, Staessen JA, Grodzicki T, Pocock S, Boutitie F et al (2002) Pulsatile blood pressure component as predictor of mortality in hypertension: a meta-analysis of clinical trial control groups. J Hypertens 20(1):145–151

GBD 2017 Disease and Injury Incidence and Prevalence Collaborators (2018) Global, regional, and national incidence, prevalence, and years lived with disability for 354 diseases and injuries for 195 countries and territories, 1990–2017: a systematic analysis for the Global Burden of Disease Study 2017. Lancet 392 (10159):1789–1858

Giovannini S, Onder G, Liperoti R, Russo A, Carter C, Capoluongo E et al (2011) Interleukin-6, C-reactive protein, and tumor necrosis factor-alpha as predictors of mortality in frail, community-living elderly individuals. J Am Geriatr Soc 59(9):1679–1685

Guasch-Ferré M, Salas-Salvadó J, Ros E, Estruch R, Corella D, Fitó M et al (2017) The PREDIMED trial, Mediterranean diet and health outcomes: How strong is the evidence? Nutr Metab Cardiovasc Dis. 27 (7):624–632

Hanlon P, Nicholl BI, Jani BD, Lee D, McQueenie R, Mair FS (2018) Frailty and pre-frailty in middle-aged and older adults and its association with multimorbidity and mortality: a prospective analysis of 493 737 UK Biobank participants. Lancet Public Health 3(7): e323–e332

Higashi Y, Sukhanov S, Shai SY, Danchuk S, Tang R, Snarski P et al (2016) Insulin-like growth factor-1 receptor deficiency in macrophages accelerates atherosclerosis and induces an unstable plaque phenotype in apolipoprotein E-deficient mice. Circulation 133(23):2263–2278

Hou H, Wang C, Sun F, Zhao L, Dun A, Sun Z (2015) Association of interleukin-6 gene polymorphism with coronary artery disease: an updated systematic review and cumulative meta-analysis. Inflamm Res 64 (9):707–720

Hubbard RE, Lang IA, Llewellyn DJ, Rockwood K (2010) Frailty, body mass index, and abdominal obesity in older people. J Gerontol A Biol Sci Med Sci 65(4):377–381

Jadczak AD, Makwana N, Luscombe-Marsh N, Visvanathan R, Schultz TJ (2018) Effectiveness of exercise interventions on physical function in community-dwelling frail older people: an umbrella review of systematic reviews. JBI Database System Rev Implement Rep 16(3):752–775

Jeck WR, Siebold AP, Sharpless NE (2012) Review: a meta-analysis of GWAS and age-associated diseases. Aging Cell 11(5):727–731

Johnson SC, Dong X, Vijg J, Suh Y (2015) Genetic evidence for common pathways in human age-related diseases. Aging Cell 14(5):809–817

Jylhä M, Paavilainen P, Lehtimäki T, Goebeler S, Karhunen PJ, Hervonen A et al (2007) Interleukin-1 receptor antagonist, interleukin-6, and C-reactive protein as predictors of mortality in nonagenarians: the vitality 90 + study. J Gerontol A Biol Sci Med Sci 62(9):1016–1021

Kachur S, Chongthammakun V, Lavie CJ, De Schutter A, Arena R, Milani RV et al (2017) Impact of cardiac rehabilitation and exercise training programs in coronary heart disease. Prog Cardiovasc Dis 60(1):103–114

Khan H, Kalogeropoulos AP, Georgiopoulou VV, Newman AB, Harris TB, Rodondi N et al (2013) Frailty and risk for heart failure in older adults: the health, aging, and body composition study. Am Heart J 166 (5):887–894

Korada SKC, Zhao D, Tibuakuu M, Brown TT, Jacobson LP, Guallar E et al (2017) Frailty and subclinical coronary atherosclerosis: the multicenter AIDS Cohort Study (MACS). Atherosclerosis 266:240–247

Korf ES, White LR, Scheltens P, Launer LJ (2004) Midlife blood pressure and the risk of hippocampal atrophy: the Honolulu Asia Aging Study. Hypertension 44(1):29–34

Lahey R, Khan SS (2018) Trends in obesity and risk of cardiovascular disease. Curr Epidemiol Rep. 5 (3):243–251

Lana A, Valdés-Bécares A, Buño A, Rodríguez-Artalejo F, Lopez-Garcia E (2017) Serum Leptin concentration is associated with incident frailty in older adults. Aging Dis. 8(2):240–249

Landi F, Calvani R, Picca A, Tosato M, D'Angelo E, Martone AM et al (2018) Relationship between cardiovascular health metrics and physical performance in community-living people: Results from the Longevity check-up (Lookup) 7 + project. Sci Rep. 8 (1):16353

Launer LJ, Masaki K, Petrovitch H, Foley D, Havlik RJ (1995) The association between midlife blood pressure levels and late-life cognitive function. The Honolulu-Asia Aging Study. JAMA 274(23):1846–1851

Lavie CJ, Milani RV, Ventura HO (2009) Obesity and cardiovascular disease: risk factor, paradox, and impact of weight loss. J Am Coll Cardiol 53 (21):1925–1932

Lin CH, Chou CY, Liu CS, Huang CY, Li TC, Lin CC (2015) Association between frailty and subclinical peripheral vascular disease in a community-dwelling geriatric population: Taichung Community Health Study for Elders. Geriatr Gerontol Int 15(3):261–267

Melzer D, Frayling TM, Murray A, Hurst AJ, Harries LW, Song H et al (2007) A common variant of the p16INK4a genetic region is associated with physical function in older people. Mech Ageing Dev 128(5–6):370–377

Menke A, Casagrande S, Geiss L, Cowie CC (2015) Prevalence of and trends in diabetes among adults in the United States, 1988–2012. JAMA 314(10):1021–1029

Messerli FH, Williams B, Ritz E (2007) Essential hypertension. Lancet 370(9587):591–603

Moreira VG, Lourenço RA (2013) Prevalence and factors associated with frailty in an older population from the city of Rio de Janeiro, Brazil: the FIBRA-RJ Study. Clinics (Sao Paulo) 68(7):979–985

Nordell AD, McKenna M, Borges ÁH, Duprez D, Neuhaus J, Neaton JD (2014) Severity of cardiovascular disease outcomes among patients with HIV is related to markers of inflammation and coagulation. J Am Heart Assoc. 3(3):e000844

Nouvenne A, Ticinesi A, Lauretani F, Maggio M, Lippi G, Prati B et al (2016) The prognostic value of high-sensitivity C-reactive protein and prealbumin for short-term mortality in acutely hospitalized multimorbid elderly patients: a prospective cohort study. J Nutr Health Aging 20(4):462–468

O'Donnell MJ, Xavier D, Liu L, Zhang H, Chin SL, Rao-Melacini P, Rangarajan S et al (2010) Risk factors for ischaemic and intracerebral haemorrhagic stroke in 22 countries (the INTERSTROKE study): a case-control study. Lancet 376(9735):112–123

Orkaby AR, Lunetta KL, Sun FJ, Driver JA, Benjamin EJ, Hamburg NM et al (2019) Cross-sectional association of frailty and arterial stiffness in community-dwelling older adults: the Framingham heart study. J Gerontol A Biol Sci Med Sci 74(3):373–379

Piepoli MF, Hoes AW, Agewall S, Albus C, Brotons C, Catapano AL et al (2016) 2016 European guidelines on cardiovascular disease prevention in clinical practice: the sixth joint task force of the European Society of Cardiology and other societies on cardiovascular disease prevention in clinical practice (constituted by representatives of 10 societies and by invited experts) Developed with the special contribution of the European Association for Cardiovascular Prevention & Rehabilitation (EACPR). Eur Heart J 37(29):2315–2381

Piotrowicz K, Prejbisz A, Klocek M, Topór-Mądry R, Szczepaniak P, Kawecka-Jaszcz K et al (2016) Subclinical mood and cognition impairments and blood pressure control in a large cohort of elderly hypertensives. J Am Med Dir Assoc 17(9):864.e17–22

Piotrowicz K, Parnicka A, Mielimąka M, Walczewska J, Falisz K, Skalska A et al (2018) Are all the former Siberian deportees with posttraumatic stress disorder patients at risk for unsuccessful aging? Int J Geriatr Psychiatry 33(4):671–672

Pischon T, Boeing H, Hoffmann K, Bergmann M, Schulze MB, Overvad K et al (2008) General and abdominal adiposity and risk of death in Europe. N Engl J Med 359(20):2105–2120

Polidoro A, Stefanelli F, Ciacciarelli M, Pacelli A, Di Sanzo D, Alessandri C (2013) Frailty in patients affected by atrial fibrillation. Arch Gerontol Geriatr 57 (3):325–327

Puzianowska-Kuźnicka M, Owczarz M, Wieczorowska-Tobis K, Nadrowski P, Chudek J, Slusarczyk P et al (2016) Interleukin-6 and C-reactive protein, successful aging, and mortality: the PolSenior study. Immun Ageing 13:21

Ramsay SE, Arianayagam DS, Whincup PH, Lennon LT, Cryer J, Papacosta AO et al (2015) Cardiovascular risk profile and frailty in a population-based study of older British men. Heart 101(8):616–622

Ravindrarajah R, Hazra NC, Hamada S, Charlton J, Jackson SHD, Dregan A et al (2017) Systolic blood pressure trajectory, frailty, and all-cause mortality >80 years of age: cohort study using electronic health records. Circulation 135(24):2357–2368

Reiner AP, Aragaki AK, Gray SL, Wactawski-Wende J, Cauley JA, Cochrane BB et al (2009) Inflammation and thrombosis biomarkers and incident frailty in postmenopausal women. Am J Med 122(10):947–954

Ridker PM, Hennekens CH, Buring JE, Rifai N (2000) C-reactive protein and other markers of inflammation in the prediction of cardiovascular disease in women. N Engl J Med 342(12):836–843

Rogers NT, Marshall A, Roberts CH, Demakakos P, Steptoe A, Scholes S (2017) Physical activity and trajectories of frailty among older adults: evidence from the English Longitudinal Study of Ageing. PLoS ONE 12(2):e0170878

Romero-Ortuno R, Fouweather T, Jagger C (2014) Cross-national disparities in sex differences in life expectancy with and without frailty. Age Ageing 43 (2):222–228

Sanchis J, Bonanad C, Ruiz V, Fernández J, García-Blas S, Mainar L et al (2014) Frailty and other geriatric conditions for risk stratification of older patients with acute coronary syndrome. Am Heart J 168(5):784–791

Saum KU, Dieffenbach AK, Jansen EH, Schöttker B, Holleczek B, Hauer K et al (2015) Association between oxidative stress and frailty in an elderly german population: results from the ESTHER Cohort Study. Gerontology 61(5):407–415

Sergi G, Veronese N, Fontana L, De Rui M, Bolzetta F, Zambon S et al (2015) Pre-frailty and risk of cardiovascular disease in elderly men and women: the Pro.V.A. study. J Am Coll Cardiol 65(10):976–983

Skoog I, Lernfelt B, Landahl S, Palmertz B, Andreasson LA, Nilsson L et al (1996) 15-year longitudinal study of blood pressure and dementia. Lancet 347 (9009):1141–1145

Soysal P, Stubbs B, Lucato P, Luchini C, Solmi M, Peluso R et al (2016) Inflammation and frailty in the elderly: a systematic review and meta-analysis. Ageing Res Rev 31:1–8

Staessen JA, Gasowski J, Wang JG, Thijs L, Den Hond E, Boissel JP et al (2000) Risks of untreated and treated isolated systolic hypertension in the elderly: meta-analysis of outcome trials. Lancet 355(9207):865–872

Studenski S, Perera S, Patel K, Rosano C, Faulkner K, Inzitari M et al (2011) Gait speed and survival in older adults. JAMA 305(1):50–58

Testa R, Olivieri F, Bonfigli AR, Sirolla C, Boemi M, Marchegiani F et al (2006) Interleukin-6–174 G > C polymorphism affects the association between IL-6 plasma levels and insulin resistance in type 2 diabetic patients. Diabetes Res Clin Pract 71(3):299–305

Tiainen K, Hurme M, Hervonen A, Luukkaala T, Jylhä M (2010) Inflammatory markers and physical performance among nonagenarians. J Gerontol A Biol Sci Med Sci 65(6):658–663

Vasan RS, Beiser A, Seshadri S, Larson MG, Kannel WB, D'Agostino RB et al (2002a) Residual lifetime risk for developing hypertension in middle-aged women and men: the Framingham Heart Study. JAMA 287 (8):1003–1010

Vasan RS, Beiser A, Seshadri S, Larson MG, Kannel WB, D'Agostino RB et al (2002b) Residual lifetime risk for developing hypertension in middle-aged women and men. J Am Med Assoc 287(8):1003–1010

Velissaris D, Pantzaris N, Koniari I, Koutsogiannis N, Karamouzos V, Kotroni I et al (2017) C-reactive protein and frailty in the elderly: a literature review. J Clin Med Res 9(6):461–465

Veronese N, Cereda E, Stubbs B, Solmi M, Luchini C, Manzato E et al (2017a) Risk of cardiovascular disease morbidity and mortality in frail and pre-frail older adults: Results from a meta-analysis and exploratory meta-regression analysis. Ageing Res Rev 35:63–73

Veronese N, Sigeirsdottir K, Eiriksdottir G, Marques EA, Chalhoub D, Phillips CL et al (2017b) Frailty and risk of cardiovascular diseases in older persons: the age gene/environment susceptibility-Reykjavik Study. Rejuvenation Res 20(6):517–524

Veronese N, Stubbs B, Noale M, Solmi M, Rizzoli R, Vaona A et al (2018) Adherence to a Mediterranean diet is associated with lower incidence of frailty: a longitudinal cohort study. Clin Nutr 37(5):1492–1497

Vetrano DL, Palmer KM, Galluzzo L, Giampaoli S, Marengoni A, Bernabei R et al (2018) Hypertension and frailty: a systematic review and meta-analysis. BMJ Open 8(12):e024406

Walczewska J, Rutkowski K, Wizner B, Cwynar M, Grodzicki T (2011) Stiffness of large arteries and cardiovascular risk in patients with post-traumatic stress disorder. Eur Heart J 32(6):730–736

Wang J, Xu D, Wu X, Zhou C, Wang H, Guo Y et al (2011) Polymorphisms of matrix metalloproteinases in myocardial infarction: a meta-analysis. Heart 97 (19):1542–1546

Wong TY, Massa MS, O'Halloran AM, Kenny RA, Clarke R (2018) Cardiovascular risk factors and frailty in a cross-sectional study of older people: implications for prevention. Age Ageing 47(5):714–720

Yang EY, Nambi V, Tang Z, Virani SS, Boerwinkle E, Hoogeveen RC et al (2009) Clinical implications of JUPITER (Justification for the Use of statins in Prevention: an Intervention Trial Evaluating Rosuvastatin) in a U.S. population insights from the ARIC (Atherosclerosis Risk in Communities) study. J Am Coll Cardiol 54(25):2388–2395

Yoshida Y, Iwasa H, Kumagai S, Yoshida H, Suzuki T (2010) Association between C-reactive protein (CRP) level and physical performance in community-dwelling elderly in Japan. Arch Gerontol Geriatr 51(2):164–168

Yusuf S, Hawken S, Ounpuu S, Dans T, Avezum A, Lanas F et al (2004) Effect of potentially modifiable risk factors associated with myocardial infarction in 52 countries (the INTERHEART study): case-control study. Lancet 364(9438):937–952

Zhong Q, Hu MJ, Cui YJ, Liang L, Zhou MM, Yang YW et al (2018) Carotid-femoral pulse wave velocity in the prediction of cardiovascular events and mortality: an updated systematic review and meta-analysis. Angiology 69(7):617–629

Frailty as Cardiovascular Risk Factor (and Vice Versa)

6

Nicola Veronese

Abstract

The prevalence of frailty seems to be higher in people with cardiovascular disease (CVD) compared to those without, but also the prevalence of CVD is higher in people with frailty compared to robust ones. In longitudinal studies and meta-analyses dealing with the role of frailty as potential risk factor for incident CVD, we have an increasing literature suggesting that frailty increases the risk of these conditions, particularly of fatal events, and independently from several potential confounding factors. Among the domains usually included in the definition of physical frailty, exhaustion, low physical activity, slow gait speed and weakness are significantly associated with the onset of CVD in older people. However, also CVD can be considered as potential risk factor for incident frailty even if the literature is more limited. In this chapter, I will therefore report and discuss the most recent and relevant findings in this topic, of extreme importance in actual geriatric medicine.

Keywords

Frailty · Cardiovascular disease · Epidemiology · Aged · Older · Risk factor

6.1 Introduction

Frailty has been traditionally defined as "*reduced physiological reserve and increased vulnerability for poor resolution of homeostasis after a stressor event*" (Clegg et al. 2013). It is estimated that one person in ten is affected by frailty in older community-dwelling people (Collard et al. 2012), but this prevalence is probably higher in other settings such as nursing home (Kojima 2015).

The prevalence of frailty in people affected by cardiovascular diseases (CVD) is significantly higher than in people without CVD (Afilalo 2011; Veronese et al. 2017a). Therefore, increasing literature has suggested that the relationship between frailty and CVD is strict and that frail people are at increased risk of CVD, but also vice versa (Afilalo et al. 2014). In this chapter, the research of frailty as potential CVD risk factor (and vice versa) will be discussed, in the light of the current epidemiological evidence.

N. Veronese (✉)
National Research Council, Neuroscience Institute, Aging Branch, Via Giustiniani 2, 35128 Padua, Italy
e-mail: nicola.veronese1@aulss3.veneto.it

N. Veronese
Primary Care Department, Azienda ULSS 3 (Unità Locale Socio Sanitaria) "Serenissima", Dolo-Mirano District, Venice, Italy

N. Veronese (ed.), *Frailty and Cardiovascular Diseases*, Advances in Experimental Medicine and Biology 1216, https://doi.org/10.1007/978-3-030-33330-0_6

6.2 Frailty as Risk Factor for Cardiovascular Disease

Frailty is a risk factor for several important conditions in older people. In her seminal paper, Linda Fried suggested that frailty is a relevant determinant of incident falls, worsening mobility/disability, hospitalization, and finally death (Fried et al. 2001). Other more recent works have substantially confirmed the negative impact of frailty on health outcomes in older people.

The acquisition of frailty as potential CVD risk factor is, on the contrary, relatively new. In a recent systematic review and meta-analysis regarding this issue, my team and I have summarized this topic finding that in ten cross-sectional investigations, not only frailty, but also intermediate stages of this condition (commonly called pre-frailty) was associated with a higher presence of CVD than in robust participants (Veronese et al. 2017a). In our meta-analysis, longitudinal data were obtained from six prospective cohort studies. After a median follow-up of 4.4 years, frailty was significantly associated with an increased risk of incident CVD of 70% and pre-frailty of 23%, after taking in account several potential confounders, such as the presence of potential CVD risk factors (diabetes, hypertension, obesity), age and gender (Veronese et al. 2017a). The association between frailty, pre-frailty and incident CVD was more evident for fatal than for non-fatal events (Veronese et al. 2017a).

Taken singularly, some studies reported the association between frailty/pre-frailty and incident CVD events. For example, Khan et al., in 2,825 American participants aged 70–79 years, found that moderate (hazard ratio, HR 1.36, 95% CI 1.08–1.71) and severe frailty (HR 1.88, 95% CI 1.02–3.47) were associated with a higher risk for heart failure (Khan et al. 2013). More recently, we found that not only frailty, but also pre-frailty was associated with an increased risk of CVD in older Italian people without any limitation in the activities of daily living (Sergi et al. 2015). Finally, in The Age, Gene/Environment Susceptibility (AGES)-Reykjavik Study, we found that frailty increased the risk of CVD of 35%, with results stronger in women than in men (Veronese et al. 2017b). This latter study has the advantage that estimate of subclinical CVD parameters (e.g. the presence of atherosclerotic plaques in coronary arteries and higher carotid intima media thickness) were taken in account in the analyses, indicating an effect of frailty in CVD development, independently from early atherosclerosis markers.

Taken together, these findings suggest that in older people, frailty can increase the risk of CVD events.

6.2.1 Single Frailty Domains and Cardiovascular Disease

If we consider the definition of physical frailty suggested by Fried et al., we can consider 5 domains of frailty (Fried et al. 2001), i.e. shrinking, exhaustion, low physical activity, weakness, slow gait speed. The association between these domains and CVD is beyond the aims of this chapter (and of this book), but some words should be spent regarding some important results.

Exhaustion, in the original definition of the Fried's phenotype, indicates a sort of depressed mood typical of frail individuals (Fried et al. 2001). The literature regarding depression and CVD is important. In a large-scale meta-analysis of 3,211,768 patients and 113,383,368 controls, major depression was significantly associated with CVD (particularly with coronary artery disease) (Correll et al. 2017). Again, in the AGES-Reykjavik Study, exhaustion was the only Fried's criterion associated with incident CVD that resists to the adjustment for potential baseline confounders (Veronese et al. 2017b).

Low physical activity is another important aspect to consider in frailty as potential CVD risk factor. Several available studies have reported that low physical activity level was associated with a higher risk of incident CVD, but the literature was mainly limited to middle-aged subjects (Li and Siegrist 2012). In a recent study, with a 10 years of follow-up, higher physical activity was associated with a lower CVD risk in a large cohort of older people (Soares-Miranda et al. 2015). After adjustment for potential confounders, greater physical activity was inversely associated with coronary heart disease, stroke (especially ischemic stroke), and total CVD, also in people ≥ 75 years (Soares-Miranda et al. 2015).

Finally, also low physical performance level (represented by slow gait speed and weakness, i.e. low handgrip strength values) are associated with an increased risk of CVD in older people. In 3,208 older French men and women living in the community, followed for an average of 5.1 years, people walking more slowly reported an increased risk of fatal CVD of three times than those walking faster (Dumurgier et al. 2009). We have substantially confirmed these findings in a large meta-analysis in which each reduction of 0.1 m/s in gait speed was associated with a higher risk of 8% of CVD in 13 prospective cohort studies reporting this association (Veronese et al. 2018). Similar results were evident for low handgrip strength as recently evidenced in a large study regarding this topic (Celis-Morales et al. 2018).

6.3 Cardiovascular Disease as Potential Risk Factor for Frailty

Cardiovascular conditions are particularly common in older people and their consequences are of clinical importance. CVD are associated with sarcopenia (a pathological condition of loss of muscle mass that often precedes frailty) and with disability (that unfortunately often follows frailty) (Kim and Choi 2013). Cardiovascular conditions are a major cause of sick leave, and diseases of the circulatory system are estimated to be the fourth most common basis for long-term disability insurance claims (Go et al. 2013).

In older people, we have some studies suggesting a potential association between CVD and incident frailty. In the Women's Health Initiative Observational Study, people with coronary artery disease (CAD) had an increased risk of frailty during 6 years of follow-up (incident frailty with vs. without CAD: 12% versus 5%; OR, odds ratio: 1.40 (95% CI: 1.11–1.76)) (Fugate Woods et al. 2005). Other studies confirmed that the presence of CVD can worse physical performance in older people finally leading to frailty (Afilalo et al. 2014; Bandeen-Roche et al. 2006).

In this sense, in 786 women participating to the Women's Health and Aging Studies I and II, the risk of 3-years disability was 16 times higher in people with CVD than those without (Bandeen-Roche et al. 2006). A recent study in 392 older individuals, persons with CVD were more likely to experience a rapid functional decline than those without (Keeney et al. 2018).

Altogether, these findings suggest that older people having CVD are at increased risk of (physical) frailty and therefore of disability and, consequently, people having a CVD event should be routinely evaluated for the presence of frailty and disability (von Haehling et al. 2013).

6.4 Conclusion

This chapter summarized the current epidemiological evidence regarding frailty and CVD. Altogether these findings suggest a significant association between these two entities that are extremely common in older people. The research regarding frailty as potential CVD risk factor is larger than CVD as risk factor for frailty, but we need more research for understanding if reversing frailty (or improving cardiovascular function) can have an influence on CVD (or frailty).

References

Afilalo J (2011) Frailty in patients with cardiovascular disease: why, when, and how to measure. Curr Cardiovasc Risk Rep 5:467–472. https://doi.org/10.1007/s12170-011-0186-0

Afilalo J et al (2014) Frailty assessment in the cardiovascular care of older adults. J Am Coll Cardiol 63:747–762. https://doi.org/10.1016/j.jacc.2013.09.070

Bandeen-Roche K et al (2006) Phenotype of frailty: characterization in the women's health and aging studies. J Gerontol A Biol Sci Med Sci 61:262–266

Celis-Morales CA et al (2018) Associations of grip strength with cardiovascular, respiratory, and cancer outcomes and all cause mortality: prospective cohort study of half a million UK Biobank participants. BMJ 361:k1651

Clegg A, Young J, Iliffe S, Rikkert MO, Rockwood K (2013) Frailty in elderly people. Lancet (London, England) 381:752–762 https://doi.org/10.1016/s0140-6736(12)62167-9

Collard RM, Boter H, Schoevers RA, Oude Voshaar RC (2012) Prevalence of frailty in community-dwelling older persons: a systematic review. J Am Geriatr Soc 60:1487–1492. https://doi.org/10.1111/j.1532-5415.2012.04054.x

Correll CU et al (2017) Prevalence, incidence and mortality from cardiovascular disease in patients with pooled and specific severe mental illness: a large-scale meta-analysis of 3,211,768 patients and 113,383,368 controls. World Psychiatry 16:163–180 https://doi.org/10.1002/wps.20420

Dumurgier J, Elbaz A, Ducimetière P, Tavernier B, Alpérovitch A, Tzourio C (2009) Slow walking speed and cardiovascular death in well functioning older adults: prospective cohort study. BMJ 339:b4460

Fried LP et al (2001) Frailty in older adults: evidence for a phenotype. J Gerontol A Biol Sci Med Sci 56:M146–M156

Fugate Woods N et al (2005) Frailty: emergence and consequences in women aged 65 and older in the Women's Health Initiative Observational Study. J Am Geriatr Soc 53:1321–1330

Go AS et al (2013) Forecasting the future of cardiovascular disease in the United States: a policy statement from the American Heart Association. Circulation 127:e6–e245

Keeney T, Fox AB, Jette DU, Jette A (2018) Functional trajectories of persons with cardiovascular disease in late life. J Am Geriatr Soc 67(1):37–42

Khan H et al (2013) Frailty and risk for heart failure in older adults: the health, aging, and body composition study. Am Heart J 166:887–894 https://doi.org/10.1016/j.ahj.2013.07.032

Kim TN, Choi KM (2013) Sarcopenia: definition, epidemiology, and pathophysiology. J Bone Metab 20:1–10

Kojima G (2015) Prevalence of frailty in nursing homes: a systematic review and meta-analysis. J Am Med Dir Assoc 16:940–945. https://doi.org/10.1016/j.jamda.2015.06.025

Li J, Siegrist J (2012) Physical activity and risk of cardiovascular disease–a meta-analysis of prospective cohort studies. Int J Environ Res Public Health 9:391–407 https://doi.org/10.3390/ijerph9020391

Sergi G et al (2015) Pre-frailty and risk of cardiovascular disease in elderly men and women: the Pro.V.A. study. J Am Coll Cardiol 65:976–983. https://doi.org/10.1016/j.jacc.2014.12.040

Soares-Miranda L, Siscovick DS, Psaty BM, Longstreth W, Mozaffarian D (2015) Physical activity and risk of coronary heart disease and stroke in older adults: the Cardiovascular Health Study. Circulation 133(2):147–155. 10.1161/CIRCULATIONAHA.115.018323

Veronese N et al (2017a) Risk of cardiovascular disease morbidity and mortality in frail and pre-frail older adults: results from a meta-analysis and exploratory meta-regression analysis. Ageing Res Rev 35:63–73. https://doi.org/10.1016/j.arr.2017.01.003

Veronese N et al (2017b) Frailty and risk of cardiovascular diseases in older persons: the age gene/environment susceptibility-Reykjavik Study. Rejuvenation Res 20:517–524. https://doi.org/10.1089/rej.2016.1905

Veronese N et al (2018) Association between gait speed with mortality, cardiovascular disease and cancer: a systematic review and meta-analysis of prospective cohort studies. J Am Med Dir Assoc 19(981–988):e987

von Haehling S, Anker SD, Doehner W, Morley JE, Vellas B (2013) Frailty and heart disease. Int J Cardiol 168:1745–1747. https://doi.org/10.1016/j.ijcard.2013.07.068

Inflammation, Frailty and Cardiovascular Disease

7

Pinar Soysal, Ferhat Arik, Lee Smith, Sarah E. Jackson and Ahmet Turan Isik

Abstract

Chronic inflammation, which is called "inflamm-aging" , is characterized by an increased level of inflammatory cytokines in response to physiological and environmental stressors, and causes the immune system to function consistently at a low level, even though it is not effective. Possible causes of inflammaging include genetic susceptibility, visceral obesity, changes in gut microbiota and permeability, chronic infections and cellular senescence. Inflammation has a role in the development of many age-related diseases, such as frailty. Low grade chronic inflammation can also increase the risk of atherosclerosis and insulin resistance which are the leading mechanisms in the development of cardiovascular diseases (CVD). As it is well known that the risk of CVD is higher in older people with frailty and the risk of frailty is higher in patients with CVD, there may be relationship between inflammation and the development of CVD and frailty. Therefore, this important issue will be discussed in this chapter.

Keywords

Inflammaging · Inflammation · Frailty · Atherosclerosis · Insulin resistance · Cardiovascular diseases · Cytokines · Microbiota · Senescence

P. Soysal (✉)
Department of Geriatric Medicine, Faculty of Medicine, Bezmialem Vakif University, Adnan Menderes Bulvarı (Vatan Street), 34093 Fatih, Istanbul, Turkey
e-mail: dr.pinarsoysal@hotmail.com

F. Arik
Department of Internal Medicine, Tomarza Yasar Karayel State Hospital, Kayseri, Turkey

L. Smith
The Cambridge Centre for Sport and Exercise Sciences, Anglia Ruskin University, Cambridge, UK

S. E. Jackson
Department of Behavioural Science and Health, UCL, London WC1E 6BT, UK

A. T. Isik
Department of Geriatric Medicine, Faculty of Medicine, Dokuz Eylul University, Izmir, Turkey

7.1 Inflammation, Frailty and Cardiovascular Disease

The prolongation of lifetime causes to increase of elderly people population and causes increase exponentially in the number of aging related diseases as well as complications related to this diseases. Major two of these diseases are frailty and cardiovascular diseases (Ferrucci and Fabbri 2018). Inflammation is one of the most accused reason for both aging and development of these two diseases. According to this inflammation hypothesis, in the case of chronic low levels of pro-inflammatory and inflammatory cytokines

N. Veronese (ed.), *Frailty and Cardiovascular Diseases*, Advances in Experimental Medicine and Biology 1216, https://doi.org/10.1007/978-3-030-33330-0_7

released from aging organs and tissues is named as "inflammageing"; and the probability of endothelial damage, vascular remodeling impairment, atherosclerosis and insulin resistance as risk factors of cardiovascular disease and frailty is higher (Ferrucci and Fabbri 2018; Soysal et al. 2016). Inflammation occurred due to genetic susceptibility, visceral obesity, changes in gut microbiota and permeability, chronic infections and cellular senescence is a common cause of these two diseases and cardiovascular disease in frail patients as well as frailty in cardiovascular diseases is seen much more; wonders the question of whether there is a special relationship between inflammation-frailty and cardiovascular disease triad (Fougere et al. 2017). In this book chapter answer of this question will be researched.

7.1.1 Aging

Aging occurs due to progressive cell damage, deterioration of tissue functions, increased vulnerability to stressors and a reduction in physiological reserves. The mechanism by which aging occurs is not yet fully understood, but mitochondrial dysfunction, hormonal changes, impaired immune system regulation, telomere dysfunction, and epigenetic modifications are the most discussed theories (Burton DGA. Cellular senescence, ageing and disease (Ren et al. 2009; Burton 2009). Environmental factors have a significant impact on homeostatic balance (Fougere et al. 2017). For example, air pollution can accelerate aging by activating oxidative stress and inflammatory pathways (Fougere et al. 2017). Chronic inflammation is characterized by an increased level of proinflammatory cytokines in response to physiological and environmental stressors, and causes the immune system to function consistently at a low level, even though it is not effective. This continuous activity of the immune system related to aging is called inflamm-aging (Salvioli et al. 2013). In some epidemiological studies, inflamm-aging has a role in the development of many age-related diseases such as cardiovascular diseases (CVD), Alzheimer's Disease, frailty, sarcopenia, cancer, type 2 diabetes mellitus and macular degeneration (Fougere et al. 2017).

7.2 Inflammation

Acute inflammation occurs as a result of acute events such as infection and trauma. By the release of cytokines such as tumor necrosis factor-α (TNF-α) and interleukin-6 (IL-6), macrophages and monocytes become activated, resulting in a systemic response with multiple organ involvement. Thus, the destruction of microbial pathogens, tissue repair and return to physiological hemostasis can be achieved. Unlike acute inflammation, chronic inflammation does not occur for same reasons, such as an acute damage or infection, and chronically inflamed tissues continue to produce signaling that allows the migration of leukocytes from blood to tissue, disrupting the process of repair in intact tissues. Therefore, chronic inflammation is the underlying cause of many age-related diseases (Fougere et al. 2017).

7.2.1 Possible Causes of Inflammation

7.2.1.1 Genetic Susceptibility

Genetic susceptibility is considered as a factor that can contribute to the effects of inflammaging, immunocompromise and their negative effects. Both pro-inflammatory cytokines (i.e., TNF-α, IL-6, interleukin (IL)-1, Interferon-α, transforming growth factor) and anti-inflammatory cytokines (i.e., IL-1 receptor antagonist, IL-4, IL-10, IL-13, IL-33) are two important components of the immune system working in harmony. However, since cytokine dysfunction increases with aging, the immune response is adversely affected. One of the most well-defined mechanisms in immune system dysfunction is genetic vulnerability. Some single nucleotide polymorphisms (SNPs; a common type of genetic variation among people) are associated with low risk for CVD and others with high risk. For example, a functional genetic variant (Asp358Ala) affecting IL6R1 has been found to be associated with an increased risk of coronary artery disease, whereas IL-6 gene 174G/C polymorphism is associated with increased risk of coronary artery disease (Collaboration IRGCERF et al. 2012; Schnabel et al. 2011). Multiple SNPs in the C-reactive protein (CRP) gene are associated with high CRP levels and death due to myocardial infarction and CVD (Lange et al. 2006). Variants in IL genes have also been associated with non-CVD. For example, correlations have been observed between the IL-1 gene and the development of osteoarthritis and acute infection, and between IL6 gene and rheumatoid arthritis, asthma and Alzheimer's disease (Del Pinto and Ferri 2018). Although genetic polymorphisms have been shown to cause multimorbidity and frailty by cumulative effect, there is insufficient evidence to support this hypothesis at present.

Some epigenetic changes that occur with aging (e.g., DNA methylation and histone modifications) contribute to overexpression of proinflammatory genes, leading to carcinogenesis and chronic inflammatory diseases (Fougere et al. 2017). Telomere shortening occurs due to accumulation of DNA damage due to inflammation. This has been demonstrated to contribute to persistent DNA damage through replicative senescence and to further increase pro-inflammatory cytokines (Hewitt et al. 2012). Potential mediators such as micro-RNAs provide modulation of gene expression. These molecules have also been displayed to induce inflammation such as nuclear factor kappa-light-chain-enhancer of activated B cells (NF-kB) signaling (Olivieri et al. 2015). There is evidence suggesting that some micro-RNAs are associated with inflamm-aging and chronic diseases. For example, lower levels of miR-126–3p have been observed in patients with CVD and diabetes mellitus, whereas miR-21 m5p levels were higher (Olivieri et al. 2015; Olivieri et al. 2014).

7.2.1.2 Cellular Senescence

One of the biological mechanisms thought to cause chronic inflammation is the accumulation of senescent cells in many tissues. Senescence, as a response to damage and stress, suppresses cell proliferation, prevents cancer growth and contributes to optimal healing of tissues (Franceschi and Campisi 2014). Cellular senescence is caused by intracellular secretion of nearly 40 soluble molecules, so it is called senescence-associated secretory phenotype (SASP) (Coppe et al. 2010). SASP has a large number of paracrine effects that stimulate pro-inflammatory cytokines, triggering the secretion of interleukins, chemokines (IL-8 and growth-regulated-α protein), growth factors (fibroblast growth factor 2), metalloproteinases, collagenase 3, and other extracellular matrix proteins (Coppe et al. 2010). On the other hand, it has been revealed that the locations of genes that play a regulatory role in senescence and inflammation are close to one another and their SNPs play a role in many diseases such as aging-associated cancer, atherosclerosis, type 2 diabetes, and glaucoma. The strongest association was found with a variant of the CDKN2A gene encoding the p16INK4A protein overexpressed in many forms of aging (Jeck et al. 2012). With aging, the number of senescent cells accumulated in organs and tissues increases exponentially. The accumulation of senescent T cells has been shown especially in patients with cytomegalovirus (CMV) or human immunodeficiency virus (HIV) infection (Fulop et al. 2013). This suggests that one of the causes of increased inflammation in patients with chronic viral infection may be the accumulation of senescent cells.

7.2.1.3 Chronic Infections

Subclinical and clinically chronic infections continuously stimulate the immune system, causing chronic inflammatory cytokines to be elevated. For example, more than half of adults are in the latent phase of the herpes virus, Cytomegalovirus (CMV), and CMV-specific memory T cells account for more than 50% of total memory T cells in the elderly (Simon et al. 2006). CMV infections increase IL-6 and TNF-α levels and cause aging-like changes in the immune system (Derhovanessian et al. 2011). In a study of 511 patients over the age of 65 years who had been followed for 18 years, it was found that mortality was higher in patients with CMV infection and life expectancy was lower than those without CMV infection (Savva et al. 2013). Other chronic infections such as hepatitis C or HIV also play a role in inflammaging. With effective antiretroviral treatment, prolonged life expectancy and decreased complications in HIV patients indicate the close relationship between chronic infections and immune system dysregulation (Lederman MM, Funderburg NT, Sekaly RP, Klatt NR, Hunt PW 2013). The results of the study investigating the relationship between CMV infection and CVD are contradictory. However, recent studies have shown that CMV specific CD8+ T-cell response in patients with hypertension is independently correlated with arterial stiffness, and there is evidence that human CMV infection may be a risk factor for vascular endothelial dysfunction and coronary heart disease (Wang et al. 2017).

However, chronic infections, such as asymptomatic urinary infections or intestinal infections, may lead to chronic pathogen-associated molecular patterns release and thus chronic inflammation. It is not clear whether the treatment of these infections can prevent inflamm-aging and associated numerous adverse complications.

7.2.1.4 Microbiota and Gut Permeability

In recent years, the hypothesis that aging gut permeability and microbiota may be related to inflammation has been emphasized. With aging, colonization of beneficial microorganisms (e.g., Coprococcus, Faecalibacterium, and Lactobacillus) in the intestine is reduced. These microorganisms are important in maintaining the intestinal barrier, preventing the colonization of pathogenic microbial agents and preventing the pathogen-associated molecules from reaching the circulatory system (Biagi et al. 2016). Frail patients have been shown to have altered gut microbiota compared to non-frail patients. Centenarians who are considered to have aged healthily, have been found to be rich in microorganisms such as Akkermansia, Bifidobacterium, and Christensenellaceae, which have anti-inflammatory activity and have positive effects on the immune system (Biagi et al. 2016).

It was found that facultative anaerobes (e.g., Fusobacterium and Staphylococcus) became dominant in the intestines of the elderly people, which was associated with increased inflammatory cytokines (Biagi et al. 2010).

It has been shown that systemic inflammation and central obesity can be reduced with a healthy intestinal flora supported by probiotic and prebiotics, which in turn may have beneficial effects on cardiovascular system in particular (Nagpal et al. 2016). For example, patients who had been administered Lactobacillus plantarum following myocardial infarction showed a significant decrease in the infarct area and improved left ventricular function (Lam et al. 2012). Moreover, the number of studies found to be related to the pathology of hypertension, which is one of the most important modified risk factors for CVD, and gut microbiota is increasing (Tang et al. 2017).

7.2.1.5 Visceral Obesity

The prevalence of obesity increases dramatically and contributes to the increase in the prevalence of many diseases such as type 2 diabetes mellitus, asthma, cancer, neurodegenerative diseases, nonalcoholic liver disease. Localized inflammation in the abdomen, liver, intramuscular, pericardial adipose tissue and the systemic low-grade inflammation induced by it have an important role in the development of all these diseases (Karczewski et al. 2018). Visceral adipose tissue in obese patients is infiltrated by macrophages, monocytes and T lymphocytes. IFN-a released from T lymphocytes stimulates T lymphocyte migration by increasing the production of chemokines (Vandanmagsar et al. 2011). The accumulation of B lymphocytes and macrophages, which cause the release of the inflammatory compound, increases with increasing body mass index (Weisberg et al. 2003). Reducing dietary intake (calorie restriction), and bariatric surgery resulting in weight loss also reduce inflammatory markers. It has been shown that in obese patients, higher TNF-alpha is released from adipose tissue, compared to non-obese ones, which causes insulin resistance by preventing insulin signaling (Fulop et al. 2018). Weight lost by exercise improves functional status in obese elderly people, reducing frailty and preventing CVD from occurring (Zomer et al. 2016). However, it is unclear whether this beneficial effect is due to control of inflammation.

7.3 Inflammation and Frailty

The age-related decline in function and reserve may lead to a reduction in the ability to cope with acute or external stresses, which is typically defined as frailty (Clegg et al. 2013).

Proinflammatory cytokines can directly affect frailty by promoting protein degradation or indirectly by affecting important metabolic pathways (Lang et al. 2009). A direct relationship was observed between the frailty and high levels of inflammation, independent of the chronic disease states associated with increased IL-6, CRP, fibrinogen, and factor VIII (Newman et al. 2001). Nevertheless, other studies have shown that these markers do not indicate frailty in the elderly (Yao et al. 2011).

A recent meta-analysis of 23,910 older adults showed that fragility and pre-frailty were associated with higher inflammatory parameters, particularly CRP and IL-6. Both high inflammatory levels and frailty are associated with some negative consequences in the elderly, such as mortality, morbidity, high hospitalization rate, disability, and co-morbidity onset (Piggott et al. 2015).

In this meta-analysis, it was found that the association of high inflammation with frailty appears to be consistent in the studies, because both frail and pre-frail patients showed high serum CRP, TNF-α, IL-6, white blood cells, and fibrinogen levels (Piggott et al. 2015). There may be several reasons for these results. First, frail and pre-frail participants have more concurrent factors such as disability, medical conditions, that can increase inflammatory markers. Second, frail and pre-frail people (especially those living in the community) are generally more obese than non-frail participants, and obesity significantly increases inflammatory parameters (Greenberg and Obin 2006; Solmi et al. 2015; Veronese et al. 2015). Ultimately, frail people appear to have a significant reduction in the innate immune system, T-cell activity, antibody production, and an increase in oxidative stress products in mitochondrial activity, resulting in an increase in serum inflammatory levels (Hubbard and Woodhouse 2010; Li et al. 2011).

7.4 Inflammation and Cardiovascular Disease

Numerous studies have shown that inflammation is one of the causes of CVD and frailty, anemia, cancer, disability, depression, osteoporosis, sarcopenia, morbidity and increased mortality. Atherosclerosis and insulin resistance are the leading mechanisms in the development of CVD.

7.4.1 Atherosclerosis

CVD, most of which develop on the background of atherosclerosis, are one of the most important causes of mortality in geriatric patients. Atherosclerosis, which is a good example for inflammatory diseases, is a process that continues throughout human life. It usually begins at an early age, but after years it begins to appear as a clinical disease in the form of coronary heart or cerebrovascular or peripheral arterial disease (Fulop et al. 2018). Atherosclerosis begins in damaged endothelial cells that allow accumulation of cholesterol-containing low-density lipoprotein (LDL) particles, which tend to oxidize in the vessel wall. This initiates a strong inflammatory reaction that occurs with the effect of the triggering factors, including the interaction of the innate and the adaptive immune cells and the endothelial cells (Libby et al. 2011). Monocytes reach the intima layer of the arterial vessel wall where they turn into macrophages, causing the release of IL-1β, IL-18, and other pro-inflammatory cytokines (Libby et al. 2011).

In the advanced process, inflammation is exacerbated by the accumulation of apoptosis and senescent cells. Complications such as plaque rupture, plaque hemorrhage and acute vascular occlusion may develop (Colin et al. 2014). Studies have shown that high-sensitive CRP and IL-6-containing proinflammatory markers, which determine the risk of CVD, are higher in both middle-aged and elderly individuals, regardless of cardiovascular risk factors(Ferrucci and Fabbri 2018).

In the development of atherosclerosis, lipid imbalance, Heat-Shock Protein Axis, pro-inflammatory cytokines and infections are triggering factors (Fulop et al. 2018). However, just as the presence of high levels of proinflammatory substances in the circulatory system and tissues may cause diseases, inflammation may also be a reactive indicator of the underlying disease. Nonetheless, neither of these two conditions can explain the association between inflammation and atherosclerosis alone. Therefore, multiple mechanisms are considered to be responsible for the development of atherosclerosis in the presence of inflammation (Ferrucci and Fabbri 2018).

It is possible to reduce the development of cardiovascular events by controlling the immuno-metabolic events that play a role in the development of atherosclerosis for cardiovascular health protection and successful aging practices (Phan et al. 2017; Netea et al. 2016). For example, in healthy subjects with high-sensitivity CRP levels without hyperlipidemia, statin treatment is associated a significant reduction in the incidence of major CVD (Cesari et al. 2003). In another example, it was found that tocilizumab (IL-6 receptor blocker) increased high density lipoprotein (HDL) cholesterol, a cardiovascular protector in patients with rheumatoid arthritis (McInnes et al. 2015).

Another hypothesis explaining the relationship between inflammation and atherosclerosis is "The Hormetic Effect". Hormesis is an essential component of adaptability to neutralize endogenous and environmental toxins. Thus, it promotes survival by protecting the metabolism from disturbing effects. In addition, hormesis is highly conserved, generalizable and pleiotropic, independent of biological models. Hormesis can prevent the development of atherosclerosis by protecting the vascular system in the inflammatory process that progresses from foam cells to unstable plaques during aging; however, repetitive stresses make the hormonal effect harmful (biphasic dose response), which increases the likelihood of atherosclerosis occurring clinically. Therefore, hormesis is considered an indirect component of inflammation (Fulop et al. 2018). Because atherosclerotic changes occur at a certain level in the majority of elderly patients, they do not seem to be preventable, however, clinical data suggest that such conditions can be prevented in patients with fewer cardiovascular risk factors.

7.4.2 Insuline Resistance-Diabetes Mellitus

Inflammation also plays a role in the pathogenesis of diabetes mellitus (DM) or insulin resistance, which has a very important place in the development of atherosclerosis as well as CVD. DM is both a major risk factor for CVD, and one of the reasons for frailty development which increases mortality due to cardiac diseases (Cobo et al. 2016).

DM may also occur as part of a single disease or metabolic syndrome. Very closely related to obesity, metabolic syndrome is the most severe group of inflammatory processes (Ferrucci and Fabbri 2018; Fulop et al. 2018). Class 5 DM, especially in the new DM classification, is the most common form of DM (approximately 40%) and the most likely form of DM with increasing age (Ahlqvist et al. 2018). This form of DM may be related to the physiological adaptation disorder in the aging period. Considering these cases, it can be said that early onset inflamm-aging plays an active role in the development of DM in class 5 form (Ferrucci and Fabbri 2018).

Recent studies have shown that insulin resistance and lipotoxicity increase neutrophil infiltration, macrophage proliferation, and the release of inflammatory mediators that induce smooth muscle and endothelial cell activation, indicating that the increase in mediators accelerates atherogenesis (Ferrucci and Fabbri 2018). Excessive oxidative stress causes endothelial dysfunction, which allows the passage, accumulation, and physicochemical modification of lipoprotein particles into the subendothelial space (Gimbrone and Garcia-Cardena 2016). Studies have suggested that individuals with DM have a shorter telomere than non-DM and a higher number of cells with positive senescent biomarkers in their arteries, an indication that atherosclerosis accelerates and inflammation increases in DM (Aryan et al. 2018). Excessive production of angiotensin II can lead to mitochondrial damage by increasing chronic inflammation (Eguchi et al. 2018). In addition, inflammation is a risk factor for the development of DM and DM complications (Ferrucci and Fabbri 2018).

7.5 Inflammation, Frailty and CVD

Cardiac and CVD, such as heart failure, myocardial infarction, atrial fibrillation, severe heart valve disease, and stroke, increase the risk of frailty. Both cardiovascular comorbidities and frailty are influenced by the same risk factors, including low physical activity, smoking, dietary pattern, obesity, DM. Additionally, many biomarkers reflecting multisystem dysfunction are common for the two. The increased inflammation and inflammatory markers are associated with frailty and CVD (Stewart 2018). The relationship between inflammation, frailty and CVD is shown as Fig. 7.1 (Ferrucci and Fabbri 2018; Del Pinto and Ferri 2018; Sadowska et al. 2018; de Araujo et al. 2013).

High-level inflammatory markers in blood have been associated with depression, decreased physical activity, multimorbidity, decreased muscle mass, and muscle strength, all of which pose a risk for both frailty and cardiac disease (Cesari et al. 2004; Stepanova et al. 2015). Inflammation is associated with a decrease in insulin-like growth factor I (IGF1), a growth factor that acts on muscle regeneration and muscle mass, and thereby causes frailty (Ridker et al. 2000). On the other hand, as IGF-1 has a protective effect against atherosclerotic plaque development, the decrease of IGF-1 due to inflammation may also cause the development of cardiovascular mortality (Higashi et al. 2016). Inflammation adversely affects endothelial activation, disrupting muscle perfusion, which leads

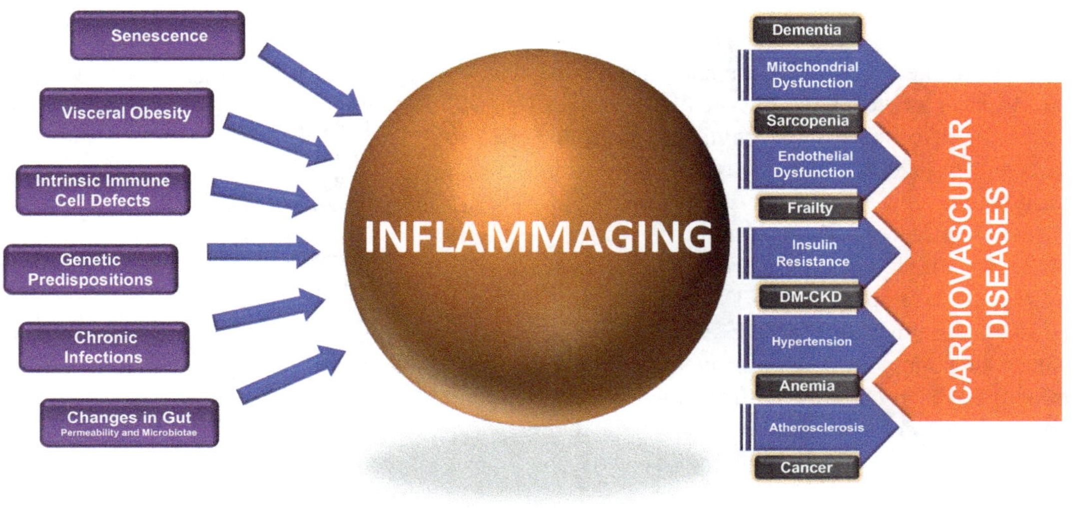

Fig. 7.1 The relationship between inflammation, frailty and cardiovascular disease

to frailty and leads to differentiation of endothelial progenitor cells, resulting in vascular damage and increasing the incidence of cardiac disease (Haybar et al. 2018; Timmerman et al. 2010). Inflammatory mediators, are produced by especially senescent cells in the elderly.

Studies show that there is a relationship between the accumulation of senescent cells and the major components of frailty: muscle strength, walking speed and mobility (Justice et al. 2018). On the other hand, accumulation of senescent cells in vascular smooth muscle cells has been found to play a role in the onset or progression of CVD (especially atherosclerosis) (Wang et al. 2015).

There are anti-inflammatory and antioxidant properties of exercise, Mediterranean diet, aspirin, and nonsteroidal anti-inflammatory drugs, and there is evidence that they can be effective in preventing both cardiovascular health and frailty-related conditions (Ferrucci and Fabbri 2018). Metformin, an antidiabetic agent, can reduce the risk of all age-related diseases, including CVD and frailty, as it is effective against insulin resistance and inflammation (Wang et al. 2017). However, further studies are needed on the subject.

7.6 Conclusion

Inflammation is one of the most important defenses of the body. There are many beneficial effects, such as preventing invasion of microbial agents or detecting and destroying tumor antigens, but chronic inflammation is associated with many age-related diseases. Therefore, the risk of CVD is higher in elderly with frailty and the risk of frailty is higher in patients with CVD. However, in the development of CVD and frailty, there is insufficient evidence on the effectiveness of anti-inflammatory treatments. Randomized controlled studies in the future will shed light on the potential utility of anti-inflammatories in reducing the risk of both CVD and frailty in the elderly.

Declarations of interest None

Declaration of Sources of Funding This research did not receive any specific grant from funding agencies in the public, commercial, or not-for-profit sectors

References

Ahlqvist E, Storm P, Karajamaki A, Martinell M, Dorkhan M, Carlsson A et al (2018) Novel subgroups of adult-onset diabetes and their association with outcomes: a data-driven cluster analysis of six variables. Lancet Diabetes Endocrinol 6(5):361–369

Aryan Z, Ghajar A, Faghihi-Kashani S, Afarideh M, Nakhjavani M, Esteghamati A (2018) Baseline high-sensitivity c-reactive protein predicts macrovascular and microvascular complications of Type 2 diabetes: a population-based study. Ann Nutr Metab 72(4):287–295

Biagi E, Nylund L, Candela M, Ostan R, Bucci L, Pini E, Nikkila J et al (2010) Through ageing, and beyond: gut microbiota and inflammatory status in seniors and centenarians. Electronic 1932–6203

Biagi E, Franceschi C, Rampelli S, Severgnini M, Ostan R, Turroni S et al (2016) Gut microbiota and extreme longevity. Curr Biol 26(11):1480–1485

Burton DG (2009) Cellular senescence, ageing and disease. Age (Dordr). 31(1):1–9

Cesari M, Penninx BW, Newman AB, Kritchevsky SB, Nicklas BJ, Sutton-Tyrrell K et al (2003) Inflammatory markers and onset of cardiovascular events: results from the Health ABC study. Circulation 108 (19):2317–2322

Cesari M, Penninx BW, Pahor M, Lauretani F, Corsi AM, Rhys Williams G et al (2004) Inflammatory markers and physical performance in older persons: the InCHIANTI study. J Gerontol A Biol Sci Med Sci 59(3):242–248

Clegg A, Young J, Iliffe S, Rikkert MO, Rockwood K (2013) Frailty in elderly people. Lancet 381 (9868):752–762

Cobo A, Vazquez LA, Reviriego J, Rodriguez-Manas L (2016) Impact of frailty in older patients with diabetes mellitus: an overview. Endocrinologia y nutricion: organo de la Sociedad Espanola de Endocrinologia y Nutricion. 63(6):291–303

Colin S, Chinetti-Gbaguidi G, Staels B (2014) Macrophage phenotypes in atherosclerosis. Immunol Rev 262(1):153–166

Collaboration IRGCERF, Sarwar N, Butterworth AS, Freitag DF, Gregson J, Willeit P et al (2012) Interleukin-6 receptor pathways in coronary heart disease: a collaborative meta-analysis of 82 studies. Lancet 379(9822):1205–1213

Coppe JP, Desprez PY, Krtolica A, Campisi J (2010) The senescence-associated secretory phenotype: the dark side of tumor suppression. Annu Rev Pathol 5:99–118

de Araujo AL, Silva LC, Fernandes JR, Benard G (2013) Preventing or reversing immunosenescence: can exercise be an immunotherapy? Immunotherapy 5(8): 879–893

Del Pinto R, Ferri C (2018) Inflammation-accelerated senescence and the cardiovascular system: mechanisms and perspectives. Int J Mol Sci 19(12)

Derhovanessian E, Maier AB, Hahnel K, Beck R, de Craen AJM, Slagboom EP, Westendorp RGJ et al (2011) Infection with cytomegalovirus but not herpes simplex virus induces the accumulation of late-differentiated CD4+ and CD8+ T-cells in humans. Electronic, 1465–2099

Eguchi S, Kawai T, Scalia R, Rizzo V (2018) Understanding angiotensin II Type 1 receptor signaling in vascular pathophysiology. Hypertension 71(5):804–810

Ferrucci L, Fabbri E (2018) Inflammageing: chronic inflammation in ageing, cardiovascular disease, and frailty. Nat Rev Cardiol 15(9):505–522

Fougere B, Boulanger E, Nourhashemi F, Guyonnet S, Cesari M (2017) Chronic inflammation: accelerator of biological aging. J Gerontol A Biol Sci Med Sci 72 (9):1218–1225

Franceschi C, Campisi J (2014) Chronic inflammation (inflammaging) and its potential contribution to age-associated diseases. J Gerontol A Biol Sci Med Sci 69(Suppl 1):S4–S9

Fulop T, Larbi A, Pawelec G (2013) Human T cell aging and the impact of persistent viral infections. Front Immunol 4:271

Fulop T, Witkowski JM, Olivieri F, Larbi A (2018) The integration of inflammaging in age-related diseases. Semin Immunol 40:17–35

Gimbrone MA Jr, Garcia-Cardena G (2016) Endothelial cell dysfunction and the pathobiology of atherosclerosis. Circ Res 118(4):620–636

Greenberg AS, Obin MS (2006) Obesity and the role of adipose tissue in inflammation and metabolism. Am J Clin Nutr 83(2):461S–465S

Haybar H, Shahrabi S, Rezaeeyan H, Shirzad R, Saki N (2018) Endothelial cells: from dysfunction mechanism to pharmacological effect in cardiovascular disease. Cardiovasc Toxicol

Hewitt G, Jurk D, Marques FD, Correia-Melo C, Hardy T, Gackowska A et al (2012) Telomeres are favoured targets of a persistent DNA damage response in ageing and stress-induced senescence. Nat Commun 3:708

Higashi Y, Sukhanov S, Shai SY, Danchuk S, Tang R, Snarski P et al (2016) Insulin-like growth factor-1 receptor deficiency in macrophages accelerates atherosclerosis and induces an unstable plaque phenotype in apolipoprotein e-deficient mice. Circulation 133(23):2263–2278

Hubbard RE, Woodhouse KW (2010) Frailty, inflammation and the elderly. Biogerontology 11(5):635–641

Jeck WR, Siebold AP, Sharpless NE (2012) Review: a meta-analysis of GWAS and age-associated diseases. Aging Cell 11(5):727–731

Justice JN, Gregory H, Tchkonia T, LeBrasseur NK, Kirkland JL, Kritchevsky SB et al (2018) Cellular senescence biomarker p16ink4a+ cell burden in thigh adipose is associated with poor physical function in older women. J Gerontol A Biol Sci Med Sci 73 (7):939–945

Karczewski J, Sledzinska E, Baturo A, Jonczyk I, Maleszko A, Maleszko A et al (2018) Obesity and inflammation. Eur Cytokine Netw 29(3):83–94

Lam V, Su J, Koprowski S, Hsu A, Tweddell JS, Rafiee P et al (2012) Intestinal microbiota determine severity of myocardial infarction in rats. FASEB J. 26(4):1727–1735

Lang PO, Michel JP, Zekry D (2009) Frailty syndrome: a transitional state in a dynamic process. Gerontology 55(5):539–549

Lange LA, Carlson CS, Hindorff LA, Lange EM, Walston J, Durda JP et al (2006) Association of polymorphisms in the CRP gene with circulating C-reactive protein levels and cardiovascular events. JAMA 296 (22):2703–2711

Lederman MM, Funderburg NT, Sekaly RP, Klatt NR, Hunt PW (2013) Residual immune dysregulation syndrome in treated HIV infection. Adv Immunol 119:51–83

Li H, Manwani B, Leng SX (2011) Frailty, inflammation, and immunity. Aging Dis 2(6):466–473

Libby P, Ridker PM, Hansson GK (2011) Progress and challenges in translating the biology of atherosclerosis. Nature 473(7347):317–325

McInnes IB, Thompson L, Giles JT, Bathon JM, Salmon JE, Beaulieu AD et al (2015) Effect of interleukin-6 receptor blockade on surrogates of vascular risk in rheumatoid arthritis: MEASURE, a randomised, placebo-controlled study. Ann Rheum Dis 74(4):694–702

Nagpal R, Kumar M, Yadav AK, Hemalatha R, Yadav H, Marotta F et al (2016) Gut microbiota in health and disease: an overview focused on metabolic inflammation. Benef Microbes. 7(2):181–194

Netea MG, Joosten LA, Latz E, Mills KH, Natoli G, Stunnenberg HG et al (2016) Trained immunity: a program of innate immune memory in health and disease. Science (New York, NY) 352(6284):aaf1098

Newman AB, Gottdiener JS, McBurnie MA, Hirsch CH, Kop WJ, Tracy R et al (2001) Associations of subclinical cardiovascular disease with frailty. J Gerontol A Biol Sci Med Sci 56(3):M158–M166

Olivieri F, Bonafe M, Spazzafumo L, Gobbi M, Prattichizzo F, Recchioni R et al (2014) Age- and glycemia-related miR-126-3p levels in plasma and endothelial cells. Aging (Albany NY). 6(9):771–787

Olivieri F, Albertini MC, Orciani M, Ceka A, Cricca M, Procopio AD et al (2015) DNA damage response (DDR) and senescence: shuttled inflamma-miRNAs on the stage of inflamm-aging. Oncotarget 6(34):35509–35521

Phan AT, Goldrath AW, GLASS CK (2017) Metabolic and epigenetic coordination of T cell and macrophage immunity. Immunity 46(5):714–729

Piggott DA, Varadhan R, Mehta SH, Brown TT, Li H, Walston JD et al (2015) Frailty, Inflammation, and mortality among persons aging with HIV infection and injection drug use. J Gerontol A Biol Sci Med Sci 70 (12):1542–1547

Ren JL, Pan JS, Lu YP, Sun P, Han J (2009) Inflammatory signaling and cellular senescence. Cell Signal 21 (3):378–383

Ridker PM, Hennekens CH, Buring JE, Rifai N (2000) C-reactive protein and other markers of inflammation in the prediction of cardiovascular disease in women. N Engl J Med 342(12):836–843

Sadowska A, Touli E, Hitzl W, Greutert H, Ferguson SJ, Wuertz-Kozak K et al (2018) Inflammaging in cervical and lumbar degenerated intervertebral discs: analysis of proinflammatory cytokine and TRP channel expression. Eur Spine J 27(3):564–577

Salvioli S, Monti D, Lanzarini C, Conte M, Pirazzini C, Bacalini MG et al (2013) Immune system, cell senescence, aging and longevity–inflammaging reappraised. Curr Pharm Des 19(9):1675–1679

Savva GM, Pachnio A, Kaul B, Morgan K, Huppert FA, Brayne C, Moss PAH et al (2013) Cytomegalovirus infection is associated with increased mortality in the older population. Electronic, 1474–9726

Schnabel RB, Kerr KF, Lubitz SA, Alkylbekova EL, Marcus GM, Sinner MF et al (2011) Large-scale candidate gene analysis in whites and African Americans identifies IL6R polymorphism in relation to atrial fibrillation: the National Heart, Lung, and Blood Institute's Candidate Gene Association Resource (CARe) project. Circ Cardiovasc Genet. 4(5):557–564

Simon CO, Holtappels R, Tervo HM, Bohm V, Daubner T, Oehrlein-Karpi SA et al (2006) CD8 T cells control cytomegalovirus latency by epitope-specific sensing of transcriptional reactivation. J Virol 80 (21):10436–10456

Solmi M, Veronese N, Favaro A, Santonastaso P, Manzato E, Sergi G et al (2015) Inflammatory cytokines and anorexia nervosa: A meta-analysis of cross-sectional and longitudinal studies. Psychoneuroendocrinology 51:237–252

Soysal P, Stubbs B, Lucato P, Luchini C, Solmi M, Peluso R et al (2016) Inflammation and frailty in the elderly: a systematic review and meta-analysis. Ageing Res Rev 31:1–8

Stepanova M, Rodriguez E, Birerdinc A, Baranova A (2015) Age-independent rise of inflammatory scores may contribute to accelerated aging in multi-morbidity. Oncotarget 6(3):1414–1421

Stewart R (2018) Cardiovascular disease and frailty: what are the mechanistic links? Clin Chem

Tang WH, Kitai T, Hazen SL (2017) Gut Microbiota in cardiovascular health and disease. Circ Res 120 (7):1183–1196

Timmerman KL, Lee JL, Fujita S, Dhanani S, Dreyer HC, Fry CS et al (2010) Pharmacological vasodilation improves insulin-stimulated muscle protein anabolism but not glucose utilization in older adults. Diabetes 59 (11):2764–2771

Vandanmagsar B, Youm YH, Ravussin A, Galgani JE, Stadler K, Mynatt RL et al (2011) The NLRP3 inflammasome instigates obesity-induced inflammation and insulin resistance. Nat Med 17(2):179–188

Veronese N, Cereda E, Solmi M, Fowler SA, Manzato E, Maggi S et al (2015) Inverse relationship between body mass index and mortality in older nursing home residents: a meta-analysis of 19,538 elderly subjects. Obes Rev Off J Int Assoc Study Obes 16(11):1001–1015

Wang J, Uryga AK, Reinhold J, Figg N, Baker L, Finigan A et al (2015) Vascular Smooth muscle cell senescence promotes atherosclerosis and features of plaque vulnerability. Circulation 132(20):1909–1919

Wang H, Peng G, Bai J, He B, Huang K, Hu X et al (2017) Cytomegalovirus infection and relative risk of cardiovascular disease (Ischemic Heart Disease, Stroke, and Cardiovascular Death): a meta-analysis of prospective studies up to 2016. J Am Heart Assoc 6 (7)

Wang CP, Lorenzo C, Habib SL, Jo B, Espinoza SE (2017b) Differential effects of metformin on age related comorbidities in older men with type 2 diabetes. J Diabetes Complications 31(4):679–686

Weisberg SP, McCann D, Desai M, Rosenbaum M, Leibel RL, Ferrante AW Jr (2003) Obesity is associated with macrophage accumulation in adipose tissue. J Clin Investig 112(12):1796–1808

Yao X, Li H, Leng SX (2011) Inflammation and immune system alterations in frailty. Clin Geriatr Med 27 (1):79–87

Zomer E, Gurusamy K, Leach R, Trimmer C, Lobstein T, Morris S et al (2016) Interventions that cause weight loss and the impact on cardiovascular risk factors: a systematic review and meta-analysis. Obes Rev Off J Int Assoc Study Obes 17(10):1001–1011

Oxidative Stress, Frailty and Cardiovascular Diseases: Current Evidence

8

Izabella Uchmanowicz

Abstract

The aim of this chapter is to review the results of recent studies analyzing the role of oxidative stress and systemic inflammation as potential contributors to frailty and CVD, and to explain a possible pathogenic relationship between the latter two conditions. Available evidence suggests that frail patients have elevated levels of oxidative stress biomarkers and proinflammatory cytokines, as well as with reduced concentrations of endogenous antioxidants. This implies that oxidative stress and systemic inflammation might play a role in the pathogenesis of frailty, but an underlying mechanism of this relationship is still mostly hypothetical. Oxidative stress and systemic inflammation are also involved in the pathogenesis of CVD. Cardiovascular conditions are established risk factor for frailty and in turn, presence of frailty constitutes an unfavorable prognostic factor in cardiac patients. Finally, some cardiovascular risk factors, such as lack of physical activity, smoking, obesity and inappropriate diet, are also involved in the etiology of oxidative stress, chronic inflammation and frailty. This complex interplay between intrinsic and extrinsic elements should be considered during holistic management of older persons with frailty and/or cardiovascular conditions.

Keywords

Oxidative stress · Reactive oxygen species · Antioxidants · Biomarkers · Physical frailty · Cognitive frailty · Frailty syndrome · Cardiovascular diseases · Inflammation

8.1 Introduction

In the era of increasing life expectancy in developed countries, a growing attention is paid to health-related quality of life in the elderly. Aging is associated with a decline of physical and cognitive reserves, and as a result, even the quality of life in older persons without any evident disease entities is worse than in younger individuals. Based on this observation, a concept of frailty has been developed as a clinically recognizable state of increased vulnerability resulting from aging-associated decline in reserve and function across multiple physiologic systems and contributing to worse ability to cope with both everyday and acute stressors (Xue 2011).

Aging is known to be a consequence of cellular damage (Pinto and Moraes 2015), which eventually contributes to organ failure and mortality (Soysal et al. 2017). The progressive loss of tissue and organ function over time was shown to be associated with systemic inflammation and

I. Uchmanowicz (✉)
Faculty of Health Sciences, Wroclaw Medical University, Wrocław, Poland
e-mail: izabella.uchmanowicz@umed.wroc.pl

N. Veronese (ed.), *Frailty and Cardiovascular Diseases*, Advances in Experimental Medicine and Biology 1216, https://doi.org/10.1007/978-3-030-33330-0_8

accumulation of oxidative damage (Crowe et al. 2016). This refers also to the heart and vessels, and CVD are the main cause of morbidity and mortality in developed countries.

Plausibly oxidative stress and systemic inflammation might also play a role in the development of frailty. However, available evidence in this matter is limited and inconclusive, especially with regards to oxidative stress, the biomarkers of which are not routinely determined in geriatric practice. To make the picture even more complicated, CVD are an established risk factor for frailty, and the latter is associated with worse prognosis in CVD (Stewart 2018). Hence, systemic inflammation and oxidative stress seem to predispose to both CVD and frailty and these two entities are apparently interrelated.

In this chapter, we review the results of recent studies analyzing the role of oxidative stress and systemic inflammation as potential contributors to frailty and CVD and explain a pathogenic relationship between the latter two.

8.2 Mechanisms and Markers of Oxidative Stress

Oxidative stress is a consequence of disruption in a prooxidant-antioxidant balance and resultant accumulation of reactive oxygen species (ROS) (Soysal et al. 2017). ROS are highly reactive atoms or molecules having at least one unpaired electron in their external shell, formed as a result of interaction between oxygen and some elements (Chandrasekaran et al. 2017). ROS may originate from both endogenous and exogeneous sources (Liguori et al. 2018). Endogenous ROS are products of some enzymes, specifically nicotinamide adenine dinucleotide phosphate oxidase, myeloperoxidase, lipoxygenase and angiotensin II (Salisbury and Bronas 2015). Exogenous sources of ROS include polluted air or water, tobacco, alcohol, heavy or transition metals, some drugs, industrial solvents, radiation and thermally processed foods (Phaniendra et al. 2015). Regardless their source, ROS cause oxidative modifications of major cellular macromolecules: proteins, lipids and nucleic acids, which results in functional and structural alterations of the cells (Salisbury and Bronas 2015).

Under physiological conditions, the harmful effects of ROS are counterbalanced by endogenous and exogenous antioxidants (Liguori et al. 2018). The group of endogenous antioxidants includes enzymes that convert ROS into nontoxic forms (superoxide dismutase, catalase and glutathione peroxidase) and non-enzymatic compounds that interact with ROS terminating the free radical chain reactions (bilirubin, alpha-tocopherol, beta-carotene, albumins and uric acid) (Birben et al. 2012; Wu et al. 2013). Antioxidants, e.g. vitamin C, vitamin E, phenolic compounds, selenium, zinc, etc., may also be provided from exogenous sources, e.g. with diet (Salisbury and Bronas 2015).

Presence and severity of oxidative stress can be determined with various biomarkers, usually determined in plasma and urine (Liguori et al. 2018). The biomarkers of oxidative stress can be divided into several groups (Frijhoff et al. 2015): (1) ROS-induced modifications, such as protein carbonyl (PC), a product of oxidative modification of proteins, oxidized low-density lipoproteins (oxLDL), reactive aldehydes produced during oxidation of polyunsaturated fatty acids: trans-4-hydroxy-2-nonenal (HNE), malondialdehyde (MDA) and isoprostanes, and DNA modifications: 8-oxo-7,8-dihydro-guanine (8-oxo-Guo) and 8-oxo-7,8-dihydro-2'deoxyguanosine (8-oxodG), (2) markers of ROS generation (e.g. myeloperoxidase), (3) markers of antioxidant defense (e.g. thioredoxin, peroxiredoxins) and (4) downstream functional markers of ROS-induced damage (e.g. asymmetric dimethyl L-arginine, phosphorylated vasodilator-stimulated phosphoprotein). Although a plethora of oxidative stress biomarkers are available nowadays, the most commonly determined group, in both research and clinical practice, are ROS-induced modifications.

8.3 Definition and Operationalization of Frailty

The definition of frailty is a subject of ongoing debate (Abellan van Kan et al. 2010). While the experts generally agree that the core feature of frailty is an increased vulnerability to stressors caused by impairment of multiple body systems and leading to a decline in homeostatic reserve and resiliency (Bergman et al. 2007), still no consensus has been reached whether this definition should be limited solely to the physical sphere or also expanded on the cognitive function, psychological status and social relations (Uchmanowicz et al. 2014). In the absence of a gold standard, Fried et al. (2001) proposed to operationalize frailty based on the following five phenotypic criteria: (1) low grip strength, (2) low energy, (3) slow walking speed, (4) low physical activity, and/or (5) unintentional weight loss (Fried et al. 2001). Based on this operational definition, a person can be considered frail is he/she satisfies at least three of the criteria mentioned above, and pre-frail if one or two criteria are met (Fried et al. 2001). However, it needs to be stressed that the Fried's criteria, although objective and used commonly by researchers and clinical practitioners worldwide, are applicable solely to physical frailty and do not cover other important domains of this condition, such as cognitive, psychological and social frailty.

Frailty has a detrimental effect on the quality of life in the elderly. The negative consequences of frailty include multiple limitations in the activities of daily living, reduced mobility, greater predisposition to falls and disability, higher prevalence of mild cognitive impairment and depression, and deterioration social relationships, to mention a few (Uchmanowicz et al. 2014). Moreover, frailty is an established contributor of higher hospitalization and mortality rates at the older age (Soysal et al. 2017). Considering all the above, WHO recognized frailty as a target of preventive interventions (Morley et al. 2013; Beard et al. 2016). According to an international consensus, frailty is a syndrome that can be reversed or at least attenuated by interventions, and as such, it needs to be identified as early as possible (Morley et al. 2013; Cesari et al. 2016).

8.4 Oxidative Stress Biomarkers in Frailty

While a link between oxidative stress and frailty has been postulated by many authors, empirical data for this relationship originate from only a few studies reviewed below and summarized in Table 8.1.

In a study conducted by Wu et al. (2009) in a group of 90 Taiwanese aged 65 years or older, frailty status was determined based on Fried's criteria (Fried et al. 2001). Using that operational definition of frailty, 21 (23.3%, mean age 79.9 $\pm$ 5.8 years) participants were identified as frail, 56 (62.2%, mean age 76.8 $\pm$ 5.8 years) as pre-frail and 13 (14.4%, mean age 73.1 $\pm$ 5.3 years) as robust. Oxidative DNA damage was determined based on serum levels of the main oxidized nucleoside, 8-oxodG. The analysis also included metabolic markers: body mass index (BMI), waist-to-hip ratio, blood concentrations of albumins, lipids and glucose, as well as high-sensitivity C-reactive protein (hs-CRP) as an established marker of chronic inflammation. Pre-frail and frail patients were shown to present with significantly higher serum levels of 8-oxodG than the robust subjects, and a significant correlation was found between the concentration of this oxidative stress marker and the number of satisfied Fried's criteria. Elevated 8-oxodG remained a correlate of frailty after adjusting for other significant determinants of this condition: age, waist-to-hip ratio, serum albumin, hs-CRP, smoking status and comorbidities (Wu et al. 2009).

The primary aim of the study conducted by Goulet et al. (2009) was to determine whether frail elderly subjects were more insulin resistant than the non-frail controls. Moreover, the authors verified if insulin sensitivity in the study subjects was influenced by various anthropometric, lifestyle-related and laboratory variables, among

Table 8.1 Summarized results of the studies analyzing a link between oxidative stress and frailty

Authors	Country	Frailty criteria	Frailty status	Age (years)	Oxidative stress biomarkers	Findings
Wu et al. (2009)	Taiwan	Fried et al. (2001)	Frail (n = 21, 23.3%) Pre-frail (n = 56, 62.2%) Robust (n = 13, 14.4%)	79.9 ± 5.8 76.8 ± 5.8 73.1 ± 5.3	8-oxodG	Significantly higher 8-oxodG levels in frail and pre-frail groups. Significant correlation between 8-oxodG levels and the number of satisfied frailty criteria
Goulet et al. (2009)	Canada	Rothman et al. (2008)	Frail (n = 33, 61.1%) Pre-frail/Robust (n = 21, 38.9%)	82 ± 5 79 ± 5	Paraoxonase-1 MDA Antioxidant capacity	No significant differences between the study groups
Serviddio et al. (2009)	Italy	Fried et al. (2001)	Frail (n = 43, 69.4%) Robust (n = 19, 30.6%)	NA	Reduced glutathione Oxidized glutathione MDA HNE	Significantly higher levels of oxidized glutathione, MDA, HNE and oxidized to reduced glutathione ratio in the frail group. Significant determinants of frailty: higher values of oxidized to reduced glutathione ratio (OR = 1.8, 95% CI: 1.2–2.5), higher concentrations of MDA (OR = 2.8, 95% CI: 1.6–4.7) and HNE (OR = 1.5, 95% CI: 1.2–2.8). Significant correlation between the number of satisfied frailty criteria and the values of the oxidized to reduced glutathione ratio
Inglés et al. (2014)	Spain	Fried et al. (2001)	Frail (n = 54, 7.3%) Pre-frail (n = 278, 37.5%) Robust (n = 410, 55.3%)	78.8 ± 6.0 73.8 ± 4.7 72.4 ± 4.2	MDA PC	In the frail group, significantly higher levels of MDA and PC than in non-frail group. Elevated MDA and PC levels significantly associated with frailty, independent of age, sex and other confounders
Saum et al. (2015)	Germany	Fried et al. (2001)	Frail (n = 210, 8.3%) Pre-frail (n = 1,463, 58.1% Robust (n = 845, 33.6%)	73.7 ± 6.0 70.3 ± 6.2 67.8 ± 5.8	BAP d-ROM TTL	In the frail group, significantly higher levels of d-ROM and significantly lower levels of TTL. Frailty associated positively with d-ROM (OR = 2.02, 95% CI: 1.25–3.25) and inversely with TTL (OR = 0.42, 95% CI: 0.25–0.69)

(continued)

Table 8.1 (continued)

Authors	Country	Frailty criteria	Frailty status	Age (years)	Oxidative stress biomarkers	Findings
Liu et al. (2016)	USA	Fried et al. (2001)	Frail (n = 142, 7.4%) Pre-frail (n = 864, 45.0%) Robust (n = 913, 47.6%)	77 ± 6 72 ± 7 69 ± 6	Lipoprotein-associated phospholipase A2 Isoprostanes	In multivariate logistic regression models adjusted for age, sex, BMI, smoking, diabetes mellitus, CVD, cancer and chronic kidney disease, frailty associated with elevated levels of both analyzed biomarkers
Namioka et al. (2017)	Japan	Fried et al. (2001)	Frail (n = 34, 24%) Pre-frail (n = 62, 44%) Robust (n = 44, 31%)	82.3 ± 6.1 80.5 ± 4.9 78.2 ± 6.0	Diacron reactive oxygen metabolite 8-oxodG Isoprostanes BAP	In frail and pre-frail groups, significantly higher levels of diacron reactive oxygen metabolite, 8-oxodG and isoprostanes than in non-frail participants. Significantly higher diacron reactive oxygen metabolite level in the frail group than in pre-frail patients. BAP level in the frail group significantly lower than in the non-frail group
Ble et al. (2006)	Italy	Fried et al. (2001)	Frail (n = 54, 6.5%) Pre-frail (n = 313, 37.8%) Robust (n = 460, 55.6%)	NA	Alpha-tocopherol	Age- and sex-adjusted plasma levels of alpha-tocopherol decreased gradually with the number of satisfied frailty criteria. Participants with the highest alpha-tocopherol levels (third tertile) significantly less likely to present with frailty than those with the lowest (first tertile) concentrations (OR = 0.30, 95% CI: 0.10–0.91)

8-oxodG: 8-oxo-7,8-dihydro-2′deoxyguanosine; BAP: biological antioxidant potential; *d-ROM* derivate of reactive oxygen metabolites; *HNE* trans-4-hydroxy-2-nonenal; *MDA* malondialdehyde; *NA* not applicable; *PC* protein carbonyl; *TTL* total thiol level

them oxidative stress biomarkers: paraoxonase-1, MDA and antioxidant capacity. Contrary to other studies included in this review, frailty was identified based on Rothman's criteria: slow gait speed, low physical activity, weight loss, exhaustion, weakness, cognitive impairment and depressive symptoms (Rothman et al. 2008). The study included 54 subjects, among them 33 (61.1%) identified as frail and 21 (38.9%) pre-frail/robust persons with mean ages of 82 ± 5 and 79 ± 5 years, respectively. The study groups did not differ significantly in terms of the analyzed oxidative stress biomarkers (Goulet et al. 2009).

Serviddio et al. (2009) analyzed four oxidative stress biomarkers (reduced and oxidized glutathione, MDA and HNE) in 43 (69.4%) frail patients identified based on Fried's criteria (Fried et al. 2001) and in 19 (30.6%) non-frail controls, recruited among outpatients of an Italian clinic. Frail patients presented with significantly higher levels of oxidized glutathione, oxidized to reduced glutathione ratio values, MDA and HNE concentrations. No significant between-group differences were found in terms of the reduced glutathione levels. Higher values of oxidized to reduced glutathione ratio (odds ratios, OR = 1.8, 95% confidence intervals, CI: 1.2–2.5), higher concentrations of MDA (OR = 2.8, 95% CI: 1.6–4.7) and HNE (OR = 1.5, 95% CI: 1.2–2.8) turned out to be significant determinants of frailty on binary logistic regression analysis. Furthermore, a strong positive correlation was found between the number of satisfied Fried's criteria and the values of the oxidized to reduced glutathione ratio (Serviddio et al. 2009).

Inglés et al. (2014) verified whether biomarkers of oxidative damage to proteins (PC) and lipids (MDA) remained significant determinants of frailty after adjusting for age, sex and other confounders. The authors examined 742 participants of the Toledo Study for Healthy Aging, aged between 65 and 95 years. Based on Fried's criteria (Fried et al. 2001), the study group was divided into frail (n = 54, 7.3%, mean age 78.8 ± 6.0 years), pre-frail (n = 278, 37.5%, mean age 73.8 ± 4.7 years) and non-frail persons (n = 410, 55.3%, 72.4 ± 4.2 years). Frail persons presented with significantly higher levels of MDA and PC than non-frail participants. Linear regression analysis confirmed that elevated MDA and PC levels were significantly associated with frailty, independent of age, sex and other confounders (serum lipids and serum cytosolic enzymes for MDA and total serum protein levels for PC) (Ingles et al. 2014).

A cross-sectional analysis conducted by Saum et al. (2015) included 2,518 persons, participants of a German population-based cohort study of aging. Frailty was defined according to Fried et al. (2001) and operationalized using population-independent cut-off values for the physical performance measures proposed by Saum et al. (2012). Based on those criteria, the study group was divided into three subgroups: frail (n = 210, 8.3%, mean age 73.7 ± 6.0 years), pre-frail (n = 1,463, 58.1%, mean age 70.3 ± 6.2 years) and non-frail subjects (n = 845, 33.6%, mean age 67.8 ± 5.8 years). The study groups were compared in terms of the levels of oxidative stress biomarkers: biological antioxidant potential (BAP), derivate of reactive oxygen metabolites (d-ROM) and total thiol level (TTL), as well as in terms of the concentrations of CRP. Frail and non-frail participants were shown to differ significantly in terms of d-ROM, TTL and CRP levels. In an age- and sex-adjusted logistic regression analysis comparing highest and lowest levels of the biomarkers, frailty turned out to be associated positively with d-ROM and CRP levels (OR = 2.02, 95% CI: 1.25–3.25 and OR = 3.15, 95% CI: 2.00–4.96, respectively) and inversely with TTL concentration (OR = 0.42, 95% CI: 0.25–0.69) (Saum et al. 2015).

The aim of a cross-sectional analysis conducted by Liu et al. (2016) was to verify if inflammatory and oxidative stress biomarkers linked with CVD were associated with frailty in 1,919 participants of the Framingham Offspring Study, a prospective study following the offspring and offspring spouses of the Framingham Heart Study Original cohort. When the frailty criteria proposed by Fried et al. (2001) were applied, the study cohort turned out to consist of 142 (7.4%, mean age 77 ± 6 years) frail, 864 (45.0%, mean age 72 ± 7 years) pre-frail and 913 (47.6%, mean age 69 ± 6 years) non-frail persons. The pre-frail group was not included in the analysis. The relationship between frailty and oxidative stress biomarkers (lipoprotein-associated phospholipase A2 and isoprostanes) was studied in multivariate logistic regression models adjusted for age, sex, BMI, smoking, diabetes mellitus, CVD, cancer and chronic kidney disease. Frailty turned out to be associated with elevated levels of both analyzed oxidative stress biomarkers. Elevated levels of lipoprotein-associated phospholipase A2 and isoprostanes, as well as increased concentration of an inflammatory marker, interleukin-6 (IL-6), remained significant correlates of frailty also in a stepwise regression model (Liu et al. 2016).

Namioka et al. (2017) determined the levels of oxidative stress biomarkers: diacron reactive oxygen metabolite, 8-oxodG, isoprostanes and BAP in 140 outpatients with mild to moderate Alzheimer's disease. Based on Fried's criteria (Fried et al. 2001), the study group was divided into frail (n = 34, 24%, mean age 82.3 ± 6.1 years), pre-frail (n = 62, 44%, mean age 80.5 ± 4.9 years) and non-frail participants (n = 44, 31%, mean age 78.2 ± 6.0 years). Analysis of covariance, with age, sex and Charlson Comorbidity Index scores as covariates, demonstrated that frail patients presented with significantly higher diacron reactive oxygen metabolite levels than pre-frail and non-frail participants; also, diacron reactive oxygen metabolite concentration in pre-frail patients turned out to be significantly higher than in non-frail persons. Moreover, both frail and pre-frail patients had significantly higher urinary levels of 8-oxodG and isoprostanes than non-frail persons. Finally, BAP level in the frail group turned out to be significantly lower than in the non-frail group (Namioka et al. 2017).

A slightly different approach was presented by Ble et al. (2006) who verified whether low plasma levels of alpha-tocopherol, an established endogenous antioxidant, were associated with frailty in older persons free from dementia and disability. The study included 827 persons participating in an Italian population-based study, aged 65 years or older. Frailty was diagnosed according to Fried et al. (2001) . Using those criteria, 54 (6.5%) study subjects were identified as frail, 313 (37.8%) as pre-frail and 460 (55.6%) as robust. The study showed that age- and sex-adjusted plasma levels of alpha-tocopherol decreased gradually with the number of satisfied Fried's criteria. After adjusting the results for potential confounders (lower extremity muscle strength, cognitive function, diseases and factors associated with vitamin E metabolism), participants with the highest alpha-tocopherol levels (third tertile), were significantly less likely to present with frailty than those with the lowest (first tertile) concentrations (OR = 0.30, 95% CI: 0.10–0.91) (Ble et al. 2006).

As summarized by Soysal et al. (2017), 6 out of 8 cross-sectional studies reviewed above demonstrated that frailty was associated with elevated levels of oxidative stress biomarkers: lipoprotein-associated phospholipase A2 (Liu et al. 2016), isoprostanes (Liu et al. 2016; Namioka et al. 2017), MDA (Serviddio et al. 2009; Ingles et al. 2014), 8-oxodG (Wu et al. 2009; Namioka et al. 2017), d-ROM (Saum et al. 2015), oxidized to reduced glutathione ratio (Serviddio et al. 2009), HNE (Serviddio et al. 2009) and PC (Ingles et al. 2014), and two studies showed that frail persons presented with lower levels of antioxidants: thiols (Saum et al. 2015) and alpha-tocopherol (Ble et al. 2006). Only one study (Goulet et al. 2009) did not demonstrate a relationship between oxidative stress and frailty; a list of potential reasons behind this discrepancy might include small sample size, analysis of pre-frail and non-frail persons as a single group and the use of Rothman's frailty criteria (Rothman et al. 2008) instead of the Fried's criteria (Fried et al. 2001) applied by other authors.

8.5 Relationship Between Oxidative Stress and Frailty

According to the free radical theory of aging, also referred to as oxidative stress theory of aging, the progressive loss of tissue and organ function over time is caused by accumulation of ROS-induced oxidative damage to macromolecules (Beckman and Ames 1998). The exact mechanism of this process remains unknown, but plausibly, accumulation of ROS inside the cell contributes to cellular senescence, a physiological mechanism preventing cellular proliferation whenever a damage occurred during the replication (Liguori et al. 2018). The cells acquire an irreversible senescence-associated secretory phenotype and synthesize a plethora of soluble factors (interleukins, chemokines, growth factors), degradative enzymes (matrix metalloproteinases) and insoluble proteins/extracellular matrix components (Chandrasekaran et al. 2017).

Oxidative stress was also shown to be associated with many age-related diseases, such as sarcopenia, cardiovascular and cerebrovascular diseases, Alzheimer's disease, Parkinson's disease and other neurodegenerative disorders, macular degeneration and malignant neoplasms (Liguori et al. 2018; Reinisalo et al. 2015; Patel et al. 2016). However, the question whether oxidative stress predisposes to all those conditions or is a consequence thereof is still a matter of debate. Similarly, we still do not know whether the free radical theory can be applied to frailty development. Although both the harmful effects of oxidative stress and frailty increase linearly with age, the relationship between these two conditions is not necessarily straightforward (Soysal et al. 2017). To this date, several hypotheses have been proposed to explain the link between oxidative stress and frailty.

First, it was suggested that oxidative stress may lead to musculoskeletal damage, since it contributes to an increase in intracellular calcium and thus, promotes proteasomal activity and accelerates muscle breakdown; indeed, ROS were shown to trigger the apoptosis of murine skeletal muscles and to decrease myoblast proliferation (Boittin et al. 2006; Derbre et al. 2014). Hence, oxidative stress likely contributes to muscle dysfunction and the loss of muscle strength, which in turn results in lesser physical activity, a major determinant of frailty (Fried et al. 2001). However, it should be remembered that reduced physical activity may also promote oxidative stress, as demonstrated both in animal models and in humans (Bar-Shai et al. 2008; Agostini et al. 2010). Consequently, a relationship between oxidative stress and frailty might be a kind of a vicious circle (Soysal et al. 2017). According to the second theory, oxidative stress might contribute to immune activation due to generation of oxidized cellular components (Wu et al. 2009). Previous studies demonstrated that as a result of oxidative stress, frail persons may show a depletion of the innate immune system components, lesser T-cell activity and antibody production (Li et al. 2011; Soysal et al. 2016). Frailty might also be related to elevated levels of proinflammatory cytokines which are one of the hallmarks of aging and were shown to promote protein degradation and to interfere with many important metabolic pathways (Lang et al. 2009). Third, frail and pre-frail persons frequently suffer from various comorbidities associated with enhanced oxidative stress, such as CVD, stroke, dementia and diabetes mellitus (Reinisalo et al. 2015; Patel et al. 2016). These conditions, often diagnosed in the elderly, might be associated with increased metabolic rate to maintain cellular homeostasis, and hence, might promote oxidative stress with all harmful consequences thereof (Saum et al. 2015). Finally, the results of many studies suggest that frail persons frequently present with excess body weight, and obesity both is an established determinant of oxidative stress and exerts a negative effect on walking ability, a criterion of physical frailty (Keaney et al. 2003; Woo et al. 2007).

As mentioned before, nowadays frailty is not considered merely as a physical weakness, but this term is expanded also on a cognitive dysfunction observed at an older age. According to literature, oxidative stress contributes to the loss of cognitive performance in the elderly (Mulero et al. 2011). Brain seems to be particularly vulnerable to oxidative damage due to a relative deficiency of antioxidants, high consumption of oxygen, high contents of iron and prone to peroxidation fatty acids and low regenerative potential of nervous tissue (Mulero et al. 2011). Indeed, age-related memory impairment was shown to correlate with a decrease in brain and plasma antioxidants (Rinaldi et al. 2003), and the studies in rodents demonstrated that dietary supplementation with antioxidants attenuated the cognitive decline and protected the brain against the oxidative damage (Fraser et al. 2005; Muller et al. 2007; Yankner et al. 2008; Park and Reuter-Lorenz 2009). Moreover, elevated PC levels were found in various areas of the brain of persons with mild cognitive impairment (Abd El Mohsen et al. 2005; Poon et al. 2006). Individuals with mild cognitive impairment also presented with significantly higher cerebrospinal fluid, plasma and urinary concentrations of isoprostanes than cognitively normal elderly subjects (Pratico et al. 2002).

8.6 Oxidative Stress and Cardiovascular Diseases

Several authors stipulated that aging is associated with lesser tolerance of the heart and vessels to oxidative stress (Liguori et al. 2018). This greater susceptibility to oxidative damage seems to be related to a systemic decrease in the activity antioxidant enzymes and is likely a significant contributor to the development of cardiovascular pathologies (Abete et al. 1999).

The primary cardiovascular condition in the case of which the link with oxidative stress became evident is atherosclerosis. oxLDL, a product of LDL oxidation, was shown to play a key role in the pathogenesis of atherosclerosis, and some studies demonstrated an association between oxLDL concentration and arterial stiffness, independent of other conventional risk factors for CVD (Brinkley et al. 2009; Paik et al. 2013). However, although the causal link between accumulation of oxLDF and arterial insufficiency raises no controversies, it is still unclear whether this oxidative stress biomarker has a prognostic value in cardiovascular patients; for example, a large population based follow-up study, InCHIANTI found no association between oxLDL levels and cardiovascular mortality (Zuliani et al. 2013).

Aside from the overproduction of oxLDL, another driver of cardiovascular morbidity seems to be oxidative endothelial damage. Brachial artery flow-mediated dilation in healthy adults of various ages was shown to correlate inversely with the concentration of nitrotyrosine, a product of tyrosine interaction with ROS, in vascular endothelial cells (Donato et al. 2007). Also, the expression of endothelin-1, a potent vasoconstrictor synthesized in vascular endothelium, was demonstrated to be positively correlated with nitrotyrosine concentrations (Donato et al. 2009). Aside from being a vasoconstrictor molecule, endothelin-1 has also prooxidant and proinflammatory properties and hence, it has been implicated in oxidative endothelial damage (Lemkens et al. 2012). Furthermore, endothelin-1 production in endothelial cells was shown to be stimulated by oxLDL (Donato et al. 2009), and endothelin-1 overexpression is known to stimulate ROS generation by NADPH oxidase (Barhoumi et al. 2014). All those findings suggest that a determinantal effect of oxidative stress on cardiovascular system is likely a self-perpetuating process. Moreover, oxidative stress stimulates inflammatory response within the cardiovascular system, and as shown further in this chapter, proinflammatory cytokines stimulate further oxidative damage in a positive reverse feedback mechanism.

Taken altogether, those findings imply that oxidative stress predisposes to cardiovascular morbidity primarily via an increase in peripheral vascular resistance, as it likely plays a role in the development of atherosclerosis and arterial hypertension (Siti et al. 2015).

8.7 Oxidative Stress, Cardiovascular Diseases and Frailty—Common Links

As shown above, both frailty and CVD seems to be related to oxidative stress and systemic inflammation. Then, there is an evident bidirectional link between CVD and frailty.

First, CVD are an established risk factor for frailty. Most cardiovascular conditions exert a detrimental effect on functional capacity, which is inter alia reflected by lesser physical activity, a hallmark of frailty (McNallan et al. 2013; Polidoro et al. 2013). Moreover, despite many published recommendations, cardiovascular patients tend to intentionally decrease the level of their physical activity, even if not justified by the symptoms (Stewart et al. 2013).

Second, frail patients are known to cope worse with their cardiovascular conditions. Frail patients with CVD were shown to have higher risk of both cardiovascular and non-cardiovascular mortality (Adabag et al. 2018). Frailty was also demonstrated to predispose to adverse outcomes after various cardiac interventions, including percutaneous coronary intervention (Singh et al. 2011), coronary artery bypass surgery (Afilalo et al. 2017) and transcutaneous aortic valve replacement (Lee et al. 2010), also after adjustment for other risk factors.

Finally, CVD and frailty share some common risk factors and some of those factors, namely physical inactivity, obesity, smoking and inappropriate diet seem to predispose to oxidative stress as well (Stewart 2018). This complex interplay between oxidative stress, CVD and frailty has been presented schematically in Fig. 8.1.

8.8 Conclusion

Available evidence suggests that frail patients present with elevated levels of oxidative stress biomarkers and proinflammatory cytokines, as well as with reduced concentrations of endogenous antioxidants. This implies that oxidative stress and systemic inflammation might play a role in the pathogenesis of frailty, but an underlying mechanism of this relationship is still mostly hypothetical. Oxidative stress and systemic inflammation are also involved in the pathogenesis of CVD. Cardiovascular conditions are established risk factor for frailty and in turn, presence of frailty constitutes an unfavorable prognostic factor in cardiac patients. Finally, some cardiovascular risk factors, such as lack of physical activity, smoking, obesity and inappropriate diet, are also involved in the etiology of oxidative stress, chronic inflammation and frailty. This complex interplay between intrinsic and extrinsic elements should be considered

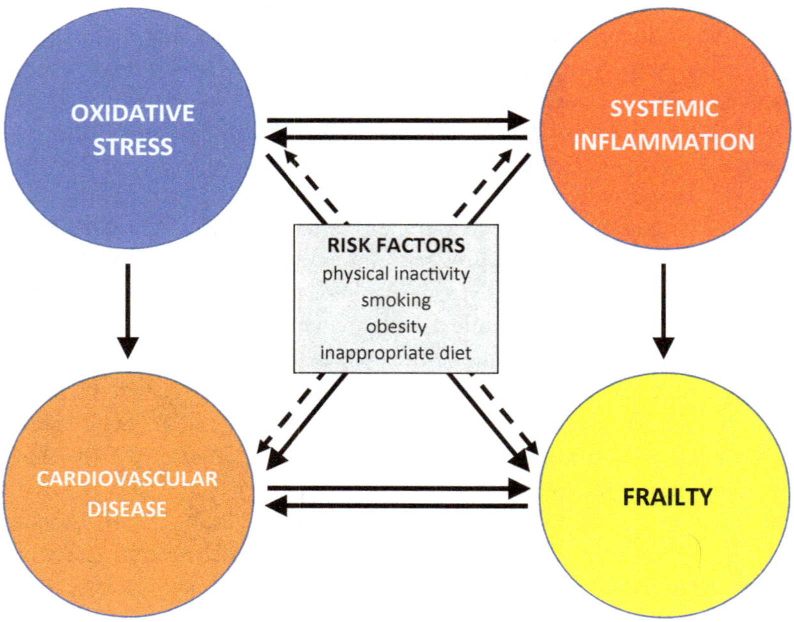

Fig. 8.1 Relationships between oxidative stress, systemic inflammation, CVD and frailty (solid lines) and their risk factors (dashed lines)

during holistic management of older persons with frailty and/or cardiovascular conditions.

References

Abd El Mohsen MM, Iravani MM, Spencer JP, Rose S, Fahim AT, Motawi TM et al. Age-associated changes in protein oxidation and proteasome activities in rat brain: modulation by antioxidants. Biochem Biophys Res Commun 336(2):386–391. https://doi.org/10.1016/j.bbrc.2005.07.201

Abellan van Kan G, Rolland Y, Houles M, Gillette-Guyonnet S, Soto M, Vellas B (2010) The assessment of frailty in older adults. Clin Geriatr Med 26 (2):275–86. https://doi.org/10.1016/j.cger.2010.02.002

Abete P, Napoli C, Santoro G, Ferrara N, Tritto I, Chiariello M et al (1999) Age-related decrease in cardiac tolerance to oxidative stress. J Mol Cell Cardiol 31(1):227–236. https://doi.org/10.1006/jmcc.1998.0862

Adabag S, Vo TN, Langsetmo L, Schousboe JT, Cawthon PM, Stone KL et al (2018) Frailty as a Risk Factor for cardiovascular versus noncardiovascular mortality in older men: results from the MrOS sleep (outcomes of sleep disorders in older men) Study. J Am Heart Assoc 7(10). https://doi.org/10.1161/jaha.118.008974

Afilalo J, Lauck S, Kim DH, Lefevre T, Piazza N, Lachapelle K et al (2017) Frailty in older adults undergoing aortic valve replacement: the FRAILTY-AVR study. J Am Coll Cardiol 70 (6):689–700. https://doi.org/10.1016/j.jacc.2017.06.024

Agostini F, Dalla Libera L, Rittweger J, Mazzucco S, Jurdana M, Mekjavic IB et al (2010) Effects of inactivity on human muscle glutathione synthesis by a double-tracer and single-biopsy approach. J Physiol 588(Pt 24):5089–5104. https://doi.org/10.1113/jphysiol.2010.198283

Barhoumi T, Briet M, Kasal DA, Fraulob-Aquino JC, Idris-Khodja N, Laurant P et al (2014) Erythropoietin-induced hypertension and vascular injury in mice overexpressing human endothelin-1: exercise attenuated hypertension, oxidative stress, inflammation and immune response. J Hypertens 32 (4):784–794. https://doi.org/10.1097/hjh.0000000000000101

Bar-Shai M, Carmeli E, Ljubuncic P, Reznick AZ (2008) Exercise and immobilization in aging animals: the involvement of oxidative stress and NF-kappaB activation. Free Radic Biol Med 44(2):202–214. https://doi.org/10.1016/j.freeradbiomed.2007.03.019

Beard JR, Officer A, de Carvalho IA, Sadana R, Pot AM, Michel JP et al (2016) The world report on ageing and health: a policy framework for healthy ageing. Lancet 387(10033):2145–2154. https://doi.org/10.1016/s0140-6736(15)00516-4

Beckman KB, Ames BN (1998) The free radical theory of aging matures. Physiol Rev 78(2):547–581. https://doi.org/10.1152/physrev.1998.78.2.547

Bergman H, Ferrucci L, Guralnik J, Hogan DB, Hummel S, Karunananthan S et al (2007) Frailty: an emerging research and clinical paradigm–issues and controversies. J Gerontol A Biol Sci Med Sci 62 (7):731–737

Birben E, Sahiner UM, Sackesen C, Erzurum S, Kalayci O (2012) Oxidative stress and antioxidant defense. World Allergy Organ J. 5(1):9–19. https://doi.org/10.1097/WOX.0b013e3182439613

Ble A, Cherubini A, Volpato S, Bartali B, Walston JD, Windham BG et al (2006) Lower plasma vitamin E levels are associated with the frailty syndrome: the InCHIANTI study. J Gerontol A Biol Sci Med Sci 61 (3):278–283

Boittin FX, Petermann O, Hirn C, Mittaud P, Dorchies OM, Roulet E et al (2006) Ca^{2+}-independent phospholipase A2 enhances store-operated Ca^{2+} entry in dystrophic skeletal muscle fibers. J Cell Sci 119(Pt 18):3733–3742. https://doi.org/10.1242/jcs.03184

Brinkley TE, Nicklas BJ, Kanaya AM, Satterfield S, Lakatta EG, Simonsick EM et al (2009) Plasma oxidized low-density lipoprotein levels and arterial stiffness in older adults: the health, aging, and body composition study. Hypertension 53(5):846–852. https://doi.org/10.1161/hypertensionaha.108.127043

Cesari M, Prince M, Thiyagarajan JA, De Carvalho IA, Bernabei R, Chan P et al (2016) Frailty: an emerging public health priority. J Am Med Dir Assoc 17 (3):188–192. https://doi.org/10.1016/j.jamda.2015.12.016

Chandrasekaran A, Idelchik M, Melendez JA (2017) Redox control of senescence and age-related disease. Redox Biol. 11:91–102. https://doi.org/10.1016/j.redox.2016.11.005

Crowe EP, Tuzer F, Gregory BD, Donahue G, Gosai SJ, Cohen J et al (2016) Changes in the transcriptome of human astrocytes accompanying oxidative stress-induced senescence. Front Aging Neurosci 8:208. https://doi.org/10.3389/fnagi.2016.00208

Derbre F, Gratas-Delamarche A, Gomez-Cabrera MC, Vina J (2014) Inactivity-induced oxidative stress: a central role in age-related sarcopenia? Eur J Sport Sci 14(Suppl 1):S98–S108. https://doi.org/10.1080/17461391.2011.654268

Donato AJ, Eskurza I, Silver AE, Levy AS, Pierce GL, Gates PE et al (2007) Direct evidence of endothelial oxidative stress with aging in humans: relation to impaired endothelium-dependent dilation and upregulation of nuclear factor-kappaB. Circ Res 100 (11):1659–1666. https://doi.org/10.1161/01.RES.0000269183.13937.e8

Donato AJ, Gano LB, Eskurza I, Silver AE, Gates PE, Jablonski K et al (2009) Vascular endothelial dysfunction with aging: endothelin-1 and endothelial nitric oxide synthase. Am J Physiol Heart Circ Physiol 297(1):H425–H432. https://doi.org/10.1152/ajpheart.00689.2008

Fraser HB, Khaitovich P, Plotkin JB, Paabo S, Eisen MB (2005) Aging and gene expression in the primate brain. PLoS Biol 3(9):e274. https://doi.org/10.1371/journal.pbio.0030274

Fried LP, Tangen CM, Walston J, Newman AB, Hirsch C, Gottdiener J et al (2001) Frailty in older adults: evidence for a phenotype. J Gerontol A Biol Sci Med Sci 56(3):M146–M156

Frijhoff J, Winyard PG, Zarkovic N, Davies SS, Stocker R, Cheng D et al (2015) Clinical relevance of biomarkers of oxidative stress. Antioxid Redox Signal 23(14):1144–1170. https://doi.org/10.1089/ars.2015.6317

Goulet ED, Hassaine A, Dionne IJ, Gaudreau P, Khalil A, Fulop T et al (2009) Frailty in the elderly is associated with insulin resistance of glucose metabolism in the postabsorptive state only in the presence of increased abdominal fat. Exp Gerontol 44(11):740–744. https://doi.org/10.1016/j.exger.2009.08.008

Ingles M, Gambini J, Carnicero JA, Garcia-Garcia FJ, Rodriguez-Manas L, Olaso-Gonzalez G et al (2014) Oxidative stress is related to frailty, not to age or sex, in a geriatric population: lipid and protein oxidation as biomarkers of frailty. J Am Geriatr Soc 62(7):1324–1328. https://doi.org/10.1111/jgs.12876

Keaney JF, Jr., Larson MG, Vasan RS, Wilson PW, Lipinska I, Corey D et al. Obesity and systemic oxidative stress: clinical correlates of oxidative stress in the Framingham Study. Arterioscler Thromb Vasc Biol. 2003;23(3):434–9. https://doi.org/10.1161/01.atv.0000058402.34138.11

Lang PO, Michel JP, Zekry D (2009) Frailty syndrome: a transitional state in a dynamic process. Gerontology 55(5):539–549. https://doi.org/10.1159/000211949

Lee DH, Buth KJ, Martin BJ, Yip AM, Hirsch GM (2010) Frail patients are at increased risk for mortality and prolonged institutional care after cardiac surgery. Circulation 121(8):973–978. https://doi.org/10.1161/circulationaha.108.841437

Lemkens P, Nelissen J, Meens MJ, Janssen BJ, Schiffers PM, De Mey JG (2012) Dual neural endopeptidase/endothelin-converting [corrected] enzyme inhibition improves endothelial function in mesenteric resistance arteries of young spontaneously hypertensive rats. J Hypertens 30(9):1799–1808. https://doi.org/10.1097/HJH.0b013e3283569c7a

Li H, Manwani B, Leng SX (2011) Frailty, inflammation, and immunity. Aging Dis. 2(6):466–473

Liguori I, Russo G, Curcio F, Bulli G, Aran L, Della-Morte D et al (2018) Oxidative stress, aging, and diseases. Clin Interv Aging 13:757–772. https://doi.org/10.2147/cia.S158513

Liu CK, Lyass A, Larson MG, Massaro JM, Wang N, D'Agostino RB Sr et al (2016) Biomarkers of oxidative stress are associated with frailty: the framingham offspring study. Age (Dordr) 38(1):1. https://doi.org/10.1007/s11357-015-9864-z

McNallan SM, Singh M, Chamberlain AM, Kane RL, Dunlay SM, Redfield MM et al (2013) Frailty and healthcare utilization among patients with heart failure in the community. JACC Heart Fail 1(2):135–141. https://doi.org/10.1016/j.jchf.2013.01.002

Morley JE, Vellas B, van Kan GA, Anker SD, Bauer JM, Bernabei R et al (2013) Frailty consensus: a call to action. J Am Med Dir Assoc 14(6):392–397. https://doi.org/10.1016/j.jamda.2013.03.022

Mulero J, Zafrilla P, Martinez-Cacha A (2011) Oxidative stress, frailty and cognitive decline. J Nutr Health Aging 15(9):756–760

Muller FL, Lustgarten MS, Jang Y, Richardson A, Van Remmen H (2007) Trends in oxidative aging theories. Free Radic Biol Med 43(4):477–503. https://doi.org/10.1016/j.freeradbiomed.2007.03.034

Namioka N, Hanyu H, Hirose D, Hatanaka H, Sato T, Shimizu S (2017) Oxidative stress and inflammation are associated with physical frailty in patients with Alzheimer's disease. Geriatr Gerontol Int 17(6):913–918. https://doi.org/10.1111/ggi.12804

Paik JK, Chae JS, Kang R, Kwon N, Lee SH, Lee JH (2013) Effect of age on atherogenicity of LDL and inflammatory markers in healthy women. Nutr Metab Cardiovasc Dis 23(10):967–972. https://doi.org/10.1016/j.numecd.2012.08.002

Park DC, Reuter-Lorenz P (2009) The adaptive brain: aging and neurocognitive scaffolding. Annu Rev Psychol 60:173–196. https://doi.org/10.1146/annurev.psych.59.103006.093656

Patel RS, Ghasemzadeh N, Eapen DJ, Sher S, Arshad S, Ko YA et al (2016) Novel biomarker of oxidative stress is associated with risk of death in patients with coronary artery disease. Circulation 133(4):361–369. https://doi.org/10.1161/circulationaha.115.019790

Phaniendra A, Jestadi DB, Periyasamy L (2015) Free radicals: properties, sources, targets, and their implication in various diseases. Indian J Clin Biochem 30(1):11–26. https://doi.org/10.1007/s12291-014-0446-0

Pinto M, Moraes CT (2015) Mechanisms linking mtDNA damage and aging. Free Radic Biol Med 85:250–258. https://doi.org/10.1016/j.freeradbiomed.2015.05.005

Polidoro A, Stefanelli F, Ciacciarelli M, Pacelli A, Di Sanzo D, Alessandri C (2013) Frailty in patients affected by atrial fibrillation. Arch Gerontol Geriatr 57(3):325–327. https://doi.org/10.1016/j.archger.2013.04.014

Poon HF, Calabrese V, Calvani M, Butterfield DA (2006) Proteomics analyses of specific protein oxidation and protein expression in aged rat brain and its modulation by L-acetylcarnitine: insights into the mechanisms of action of this proposed therapeutic agent for CNS disorders associated with oxidative stress. Antioxid Redox Signal 8(3–4):381–394. https://doi.org/10.1089/ars.2006.8.381

Pratico D, Clark CM, Liun F, Rokach J, Lee VY, Trojanowski JQ (2002) Increase of brain oxidative stress in mild cognitive impairment: a possible predictor of Alzheimer disease. Arch Neurol 59(6):972–976

Reinisalo M, Karlund A, Koskela A, Kaarniranta K, Karjalainen RO (2015) Polyphenol stilbenes: molecular mechanisms of defence against oxidative stress and aging-related diseases. Oxid Med Cell Longev 2015:340520. https://doi.org/10.1155/2015/340520

Rinaldi P, Polidori MC, Metastasio A, Mariani E, Mattioli P, Cherubini A et al (2003) Plasma antioxidants are similarly depleted in mild cognitive impairment and in Alzheimer's disease. Neurobiol Aging 24 (7):915–919

Rothman MD, Leo-Summers L, Gill TM (2008) Prognostic significance of potential frailty criteria. J Am Geriatr Soc 56(12):2211–2216. https://doi.org/10.1111/j.1532-5415.2008.02008.x

Salisbury D, Bronas U (2015) Reactive oxygen and nitrogen species: impact on endothelial dysfunction. Nurs Res 64(1):53–66. https://doi.org/10.1097/nnr.0000000000000068

Saum KU, Muller H, Stegmaier C, Hauer K, Raum E, Brenner H (2012) Development and evaluation of a modification of the Fried frailty criteria using population-independent cutpoints. J Am Geriatr Soc 60(11):2110–2115. https://doi.org/10.1111/j.1532-5415.2012.04192.x

Saum KU, Dieffenbach AK, Jansen EH, Schottker B, Holleczek B, Hauer K et al (2015) Association between oxidative stress and frailty in an elderly german population: results from the ESTHER cohort study. Gerontology 61(5):407–415. https://doi.org/10.1159/000380881

Serviddio G, Romano AD, Greco A, Rollo T, Bellanti F, Altomare E et al (2009) Frailty syndrome is associated with altered circulating redox balance and increased markers of oxidative stress. Int J Immunopathol Pharmacol 22(3):819–827. https://doi.org/10.1177/039463200902200328

Singh M, Rihal CS, Lennon RJ, Spertus JA, Nair KS, Roger VL (2011) Influence of frailty and health status on outcomes in patients with coronary disease undergoing percutaneous revascularization. Circ Cardiovasc Qual Outcomes 4(5):496–502. https://doi.org/10.1161/circoutcomes.111.961375

Siti HN, Kamisah Y, Kamsiah J (2015) The role of oxidative stress, antioxidants and vascular inflammation in cardiovascular disease (a review). Vascul Pharmacol 71:40–56. https://doi.org/10.1016/j.vph.2015.03.005

Soysal P, Stubbs B, Lucato P, Luchini C, Solmi M, Peluso R et al (2016) Inflammation and frailty in the elderly: a systematic review and meta-analysis. Ageing Res Rev 31:1–8. https://doi.org/10.1016/j.arr.2016.08.006

Soysal P, Isik AT, Carvalho AF, Fernandes BS, Solmi M, Schofield P et al (2017) Oxidative stress and frailty: a systematic review and synthesis of the best evidence. Maturitas 99:66–72. https://doi.org/10.1016/j.maturitas.2017.01.006

Stewart R (2018) Cardiovascular disease and frailty: what are the mechanistic links? Clin Chem. https://doi.org/10.1373/clinchem.2018.287318

Stewart R, Held C, Brown R, Vedin O, Hagstrom E, Lonn E et al (2013) Physical activity in patients with stable coronary heart disease: an international perspective. Eur Heart J 34(42):3286–3293. https://doi.org/10.1093/eurheartj/eht258

Uchmanowicz I, Jankowska-Polanska B, Loboz-Rudnicka M, Manulik S, Loboz-Grudzien K, Gobbens RJ (2014) Cross-cultural adaptation and reliability testing of the tilburg frailty indicator for optimizing care of polish patients with frailty syndrome. Clin Interv Aging 9:997–1001. https://doi.org/10.2147/cia.S64853

Woo J, Leung J, Kwok T (2007) BMI, body composition, and physical functioning in older adults. Obes (Silver Spring) 15(7):1886–1894. https://doi.org/10.1038/oby.2007.223

Wu IC, Shiesh SC, Kuo PH, Lin XZ (2009) High oxidative stress is correlated with frailty in elderly chinese. J Am Geriatr Soc 57(9):1666–1671. https://doi.org/10.1111/j.1532-5415.2009.02392.x

Wu JQ, Kosten TR, Zhang XY (2013) Free radicals, antioxidant defense systems, and schizophrenia. Prog Neuropsychopharmacol Biol Psychiatry 46:200–206. https://doi.org/10.1016/j.pnpbp.2013.02.015

Xue QL (2011) The frailty syndrome: definition and natural history. Clin Geriatr Med 27(1):1–15. https://doi.org/10.1016/j.cger.2010.08.009

Yankner BA, Lu T, Loerch P (2008) The aging brain. Annu Rev Pathol 3:41–66. https://doi.org/10.1146/annurev.pathmechdis.2.010506.092044

Zuliani G, Morieri ML, Volpato S, Vigna GB, Bosi C, Maggio M et al (2013) Determinants and clinical significance of plasma oxidized LDLs in older individuals. A 9 years follow-up study. Atherosclerosis. 226(1):201–207. https://doi.org/10.1016/j.atherosclerosis.2012.10.028

9 The Importance of Cellular Senescence in Frailty and Cardiovascular Diseases

Virginia Boccardi and Patrizia Mecocci

Abstract

Frailty is a complex clinical syndrome, progressively described in the last thirty years, resulting from multiple impairments across many organs and systems and characterized by a reduction in physiological reserves and increased vulnerability to stressors, as well. Cardiovascular diseases (CVDs) are a common health problem in very old populations. Age-related changes occur throughout the body and in all organs, including the cardiovascular system. Cellular senescence links age-related CVDs and frailty by many mechanisms of particular interest in the aging biology and geriatric syndromes. Cellular senescence may represent the pivotal factor with its senescence-associated secretory phenotype (SASP) leading to systemic inflammation. In this context, SASP may represent the key element in the association between aging, frailty and the development of age-related CVDs.

Keywords

Aging · Cardiovascular · Comorbidities · Frailty · Inflammation · Senescence

V. Boccardi (✉) · P. Mecocci
Department of Medicine, Santa Maria della Misericordia Hospital, Section of Gerontology and Geriatrics, University of Perugia, Piazzale Gambuli 1, 06132 Perugia, Italy
e-mail: virginia.boccardi@unipg.it

9.1 Introduction and Overview

The old age population is increasing worldwide at an impressive rate. However, while people are more long-lived, parameters of health span—defined as the years lived in health—have stagnated for years. In the last fifty years, death rates for chronic diseases have changed dramatically. Due to the reduction of many modifiable risk factors including smoking or high blood pressure, acute heart disease death is declining.

Nevertheless, all over the world, the old age population is growing rapidly and, in spite of the relative success of clinical medicine for early detection and management of chronic diseases, the gain in longevity pushed older adults in a long period of multimorbidity. A recent large population study showed that European countries would have about 21% of female and about 17% male over 65 years with severe long-term activity limitations by 2047 (Scherbov and Weber 2017). In Italian oldest old subjects (over 85 years old), these percentages will reach 49% in women and 34% in men. Thus, the goal of the modern biomedical research is to try to compress, if not eliminate, the long period of disability and to lengthen years of health.

Aging is a process characterized by a progressive decline in physiological functions, leading to an increased vulnerability to diseases and risk of death. Thus, age per se remains the major risk factor for several chronic conditions, including cardiovascular diseases (CVDs).

N. Veronese (ed.), *Frailty and Cardiovascular Diseases*, Advances in Experimental Medicine and Biology 1216, https://doi.org/10.1007/978-3-030-33330-0_9

However, aging is an extremely heterogeneous process, and three different phenotypes have been described so far: (1) normal aging (2) successful aging and (3) unfit or accelerated aging. The accumulation of different chronic diseases in the same person determines a phenotype of accelerated aging, with a relevant decline in the muscle mass as well as an increment of the basic metabolic rate (Fried et al. 2004). Thus, the loss in resiliency and the increased vulnerability to many and different stressors, which inevitably occur along with aging, is recognized as "frailty." At present, there are many operational definitions of frailty, as already discussed in this book, but recently it has been proposed as a syndrome of "accelerated aging." Briefly, as described by Ferrucci et al. (2018), frailty can be conceptualized as a construct of many overlaying dimensions. Just like to layers of an onion. The outside layer is the clinical presentation or functional aging that affects daily life and includes multimorbidity, cognitive and physical impairment. Going inside there are the hypothetical pathophysiologic mechanisms and including inflammation, anabolic hormone deficit, energy unbalance, loss of weight, weakness, neurodegeneration and poor endurance. At the hearth of this construct holds the biological mechanisms, including genomic instability, telomere attrition, epigenetic alterations, loss of proteostasis, mitochondrial dysfunction, deregulated nutrient sensing, stem cells exhaustion, and altered intercellular communication (López-Otín et al. 2013; Afilalo et al. 2014). Among them, there is the cellular senescence. Upon this model construction, frailty may be considered as the solid substrate for geriatric syndromes susceptibility. The prevalence of frailty in older adults living in community is estimated to be around 10% (Collard et al. 2012), rising to 60% in subjects affected by CVDs (Afilalo et al. 2009).

Interestingly, frailty has been implicated as a causative and prognostic factor in patients with CVDs. In CVDs, frailty is associated with a significant increase in mortality, even after adjustment for age and presence of other chronic conditions (Matsuzawa et al. 2013). However, what is the fundamental "biological link" among aging, frailty, and CVDs? Cellular senescence is emerging as a pivotal contributor and linking mechanism. In this chapter, we will review the existing literature regarding the importance of cellular senescence in frailty as well as CVDs to better define linking mechanisms.

9.2 Cellular Senescence

Cellular senescence has been first described as a natural process that limited the proliferation and growth of normal human cells in colture (Hayflick and Moorhead 1961). At present, three distinct origins of senescent cells have been recognized and well described: (1) "replicative senescence" , or cells that have reached their limit and unable to further divide (2) "cellular senescence", or cells that are blocked in the G0 phase of the cell cycle, as induced by many and different stimuli, before the loss of the proliferative capacity (3) "non replicative senescence", or non-proliferative cells because terminally differentiated (such as neurons). Interestingly, cellular senescence is not only characterized by a simple loss in the replicative capacity, but also by a series of changes in cell structure, morphology, gene expression and metabolism (van Deursen 2014). In detail, senescent cells are in a metabolically active state, that can alter the microenvironment through the "senescence-associated secretory phenotype (SASP)." SASP refers to the secretion of several molecules where interleukin IL-1, IL-6, IL-8, transforming growth factor (TGF)-β, and tumor necrosis factor (TNF)-α, have the main impact. SASP, together with the accumulation of β-galactosidase (SAβG), and increased activity of the cell cycle regulating protein p16 Ink4a, the tumor protein p53, and the heterochromatin foci, are the main biomarkers of cellular senescence. One of the key functions of SASP is the regulation and modulation of the immune system to eliminate senescent cells. Inflammatory proteins, secreted by immune cells, act in an autocrine and paracrine manner, spreading senescence via a "bystander effect," as previously reported (Acosta et al. 2013). Collectively, senescence induces extensive metabolic and bioenergetics changes in cells, tissues and whole body function (Quijano et al. 2012). The accumulation of senescent cells in tissues, organs, systems, and whole body as well, is considered as the principal underlying mechanism of aging. However, cellular senescence has a dual role, from aging progression to protection from development and growth of cancers. First, activation of the senescence process is fundamental to avoid uncontrolled cellular replication. Accumulation of senescent cells that increases along with age is the key element for tumor suppressor pathways, but it is also a promoter of tissue repair.

Nevertheless, cellular senescence has a dark side: in addition to suppressing tumorigenesis, it might promote fuel inflammation associated with cancer progression. So, if the presence and the efficient elimination of senescent cells are critical for tissue remodeling, their chronic accumulation may lead to accelerated aging. Thus, in young people, senescent cells act as a security mechanism that prevents tumor transformation but, in the old ones, accumulation of senescent cells not only promotes the appearance of a senescent phenotype, but also the generation of a favorable environment for tumorigenesis In conclusion, cellular senescence is described from evolutionary theories as an antagonistically pleiotropic process, with both beneficial and deleterious effects.

9.3 Frailty as Clinical Syndrome of Accelerated Ageing

When a stressor occurs, the organism reaction involves mainly three cellular responses (1) apoptosis (2) senescence or (3) repair. Usually, after an injury, apoptosis is activated to remove damaged or aberrant cells through controlled cell death, senescence alters cell phenotype and blocks further replication, while repair machinery properly removes waste products (as damaged proteins, lipids, and organelles). Dysregulation of these coordinated cellular responses may lead to tissue dysfunction when increased apoptosis induces organ atrophy or when the higher expression of senescent cells increases the pro-inflammatory status. The "perfect" balance among apoptosis, senescence, and repair is the key element to avoid accelerated aging. The difference between these conditions could be in the "normal or abnormal" response to stressors, that can determinate the individual rate of senescence. It may be expected that the patterns observed in normal aging among these cellular responses may be much accelerated in the syndrome of frailty.

Frailty may be considered as a clinical syndrome of "accelerated aging" characterized by weakness, weight loss, and low activity that is associated with adverse health outcomes. This is due to the loss of homeostasis that predisposes to a higher vulnerability to many and different stressors. In this context, inflammation may be considered as the systemic response to stressors. Thus, "sickness behavior"—including fatigue, loss of interest in social activities, changes in sleep and appetite patterns, difficulty concentrating and depression—may be caused by the inflammatory state linked to senescence (Dantzer 2009). Accordingly, many are the evidence showing the association between inflammation and frailty in old age subjects (Leng et al. 2011; Lee et al. 2016). Moreover, the altered inflammatory state observed in frailty may contribute to several frailty-associated diseases.

9.4 Cellular Senescence and Cardiovascular Diseases

Cellular senescence is the major contributing factor to age-associated organs and systems dysfunction, including cardiovascular, and represents the core feature of the age-related changes (ARCs). In summary, the ARCs arise from intrinsic and extrinsic causes: the first are those resulting from programmed processes, while the second is the result of experiential wear and tear and of randomly occurring, or stochastic, damaging events during life (Boccardi et al. 2017). Strongly connected to aging, CVDs are a common problem in the old age population. Atherosclerosis, heart failure, and atrial fibrillation are important cardiovascular problems where age represents the primary risk factor. Everything starts at the biological level: endothelial, vascular smooth muscle (VSMC) and cardiomyocyte cells play a pivotal role in the maintenance and regeneration of cardiovascular tissue.

Along with aging, as the result of these cellular events, the structure and function of the cardiovascular system progressively change, from the cellular to the structural and functional level. Structural modifications involve the myocardium, valves and the cardiac conduction system. The progressive degeneration and collective changes in the cardiovascular system (ARCs) along with aging are summarized in Table 9.1.

Cardiac senescence is characterized by both quantitative (reduction in the number of cardiomyocytes), and qualitative (changes in cardiomyocyte properties) alterations (Centurione et al. 2002). Molecules such as lipofuscin—a brown granular pigment consisting of cross-linked lipids and proteins produced during lysosomal digestion-, and amyloid-aggregates of insoluble fibrous proteins-, can be found in the aged myocardium (Lakatta and Levy 2003). Senescent cardiomyocytes are characterized by prolonged relaxation, diminished contraction speed, a reduction in the β-adrenergic response, and an increase in the myocardial stiffness. Furthermore, the increase in the size of cardiomyocytes contributes to age-associated diastolic dysfunction. This alteration in left ventricular diastolic function leads to the higher incidence of heart failure and atrial fibrillation in old age populations. Cardiomyocyte hypertrophy is also very pronounced in the aged heart and associated with changes in cytoskeletal proteins that may alter the microtubule architecture and the organization of sarcomeres in myocytes. Increased collagen volume fraction, higher resting cardiomyocyte tension and larger cardiomyocyte diameter are correlated with left ventricular diastolic stiffness. Also, hypertrophic cardiomyocytes require more energy by the pool of dysfunctional mitochondria. Mitochondrial dysfunction is often associated with increased production of reactive oxygen species (ROS)

Table 9.1 Cardiovascular Age Related Changes (ARCs)

Myocardial subcellular changes	The nucleus, containing DNA, becomes larger and may show invagination of its membrane. The mitochondria show alterations in size, shape, cristal pattern, and matrix density, which reduce their functional surface. The cytoplasm is marked by fatty infiltration or degeneration, vacuole formation, and a progressive accumulation of pigments, such as lipofuscin. The combined age related changes in the subcellular compartments of the cells result in decreased cellular activities such as altered homeostasis, protein synthesis, and degradation rates
Valves	An age-related increase in valvular circumference has been reported in all four cardiac valves (aortic semilunar valve, semilunar valve, bicuspid valve, tricuspid valve), with the greatest changes occurring in the aortic valve (the valve between the left ventricle and the aorta). Calcific deposits frequently are present. These changes do not usually cause significant dysfunction, although in some older adults, severe aortic valvular stenosis and mitral valvular insufficiency are related to degenerative changes with age
Blood vessels	Factors that contribute to the increased wall thickening and stiffening in aging include increased collagen, reduced elastin, and calcification. The decrease of elasticity of the arterial vessels with aging may result in chronic or residual increases in vessel diameter and vessel wall rigidity, which impair their function
Electrical conduction system	First, cardiac conduction is affected by the decrease in the number of pacemaker cells in the sinoatrial node with age. With advancing age, there is an increase in elastic and collagenous tissue in all parts of the conduction system. Fat accumulates around the sinoatrial node, sometimes producing a partial or complete separation of the node from the atrial musculature
Cardic output	The decline in left ventricular compliance provides an increase workload on the atria, resulting in hypertrophy of the atria. Cardiac output at rest is unaffected by age, while Maximum cardiac output and aerobic capacity are reduced with age

that furtherly damage cardiomyocytes leading them to apoptosis.

Age-associated cellular changes may enhance the risk of developing CVDs. Inflammatory factors -such as IL-6, TNF-α, and acute-phase proteins—are recognized as pathogenic factors in the development of CVDs. In this context, cellular senescence and related inflammation play a key role in the genesis as well as progression of several cardiovascular diseases

9.4.1 Atherosclerosis

CVDs due to atherosclerosis is the primary cause of mortality worldwide. Increased numbers of SAβG-positive vascular smooth cells (VSMCs), endothelial cells (ECs), and monocyte/macrophages have been found in the aged vessel as well as atherosclerotic lesions (Matthews et al. 2006; Minamino and Komuro 2002), reinforcing the idea that atherosclerosis is associated with premature cellular senescence. During plaque formation and progression, smooth-muscle proliferation and subsequent decline in endothelial nitric oxide synthase levels can lead to oxidative stress (DeMello et al. 2015; Kawashima and Yokoyama 2004). These alterations are strong inducers of cellular senescence, as reported in human and mouse atheroma (Wang and Bennett 2012) (Bürrig). A sequential role of senescent cells in atherogenesis has been described: First, senescent endothelial cells accumulation induces plaque initiation, which, through the SASP activation, promotes the initial invasion of circulating monocytes into the vessel wall. Also, senescent endothelial cells are more susceptible to apoptosis, leading endothelial layer "leakiness" that allow extravasation of oxidized LDL into the vessel wall. Then, accumulation of senescent endothelial cells promotes a dysfunction in signaling, such as secretion of nitric oxide (NO), driving early intimal thickening, a well known key risk factor for atherosclerosis (Zhang et al. 2002; Krouwer et al. 2012). Later, plaque progression is mediated by chemoattractant factors in the SASP, with known pro-atherosclerotic functions (Rippe et al. 2012). Finally, senescent cells contribute to plaque destabilization and more prone to the rupture and defined "vulnerable" plaques that lead to acute complications, such as stroke as well as myocardial infarction.

9.4.2 Heart Failure

Heart failure (HF) is another typical age-associated disease. It is the last stage of many CVDs resulting in a progressive weakening of the global cardiac function, related to the dysfunctional hypertrophic and apoptotic state of terminally differentiated cardiac myocytes (Leri et al. 2003). The mechanism of HF is still not completely identified and understood, although there is strong evidence of cardiac endothelial cell senescence in its onset and progression. Heart disease associated with hypertension represents the main causes of HF. When cardiac tissue is chronically exposed to pressure overload, hypertrophy occurs as an adaptive response to maintain the systolic function. It has been demonstrated that increased cardiac expression of the tumor protein p53, which promotes cellular senescence, leads to cardiac dysfunction as shown in a murine model of hypertension (Katsuumi et al. 2018). p53 signaling activation in vascular endothelial cells leads to senescence, SASP and next cardiac remodeling (Yoshida et al. 2015).

9.4.3 Atrial Fibrillation

Atrial fibrillation (AF) is a high prevalent condition in the old population, and its incidence is expected to even double in the next twenty years (Kotecha and Piccini 2015). It is generally known recognized that fibrosis contributes to atrial structural remodeling, the structural base for development of AF (Kotecha and Piccini 2015). However, the underlying mechanisms of fibrosis in AF remain unclear. According to a recent study by Meyer et al. (2016), cardiac fibroblasts (CFs) senescence play an essential anti-fibrotic role as shown in a murine model. Similar results have been obtained from tissues of heart biopsies from patients affected by idiopathic cardiomyopathy, that showed a positive and significant relationship between senescence and fibrosis. These findings strongly support the concept that senescence is associated with atrial fibrosis in the development of AF (Meyer et al. 2016).

9.5 Frailty and Cardiovascular Diseases Linked by Cellular Senescence

Since frailty and CVDs share common aspects (Soysal et al. 2016), it is reasonable to conclude that frailty represents a significant risk factor for CVDs. A large epidemiologic study showed the association of frailty with subclinical CVDs (Newman et al. 2001). In the Cardiovascular Health Study, the prevalence of HF resulted eight times higher in frail patients than in non-frail subjects (Newman et al. 2001). Frailty might predispose cardiac tissue to damage by reducing resistance to many stressors including myocardial ischemia, pressure or volume overload as well as rhythm alterations. Among several tissues and organ systems, cardiovascular dysfunction is more frequently associated with the frail phenotype (Nadruz et al. 2017). Although the pathways leading to CVDs and frailty are complex, both are linked to chronic low-grade inflammation. Circulating inflammatory markers including neutrophils, monocytes, high-sensitivity C-reactive protein, and interleukin-6 (IL-6) are increased in CVDs and frailty (Cesari et al. 2004; Leng et al. 2009). High inflammation levels correspond to higher markers of thrombosis that could play an additional role in CVDs onset. In this context, cellular senescence exhibit a distinctive pattern of proteins expression for the induction of replicative senescence in vitro (Kortlever et al. 2006). In addition to sharing causal pathways, CVDs has been shown to contribute themselves in frailty susceptibility (Dumurgier et al. 2009).

9.6 Conclusions

In conclusion, it is possible to conceive a conceptual framework where cellular senescence links inflammation and cardiovascular diseases (Fig. 9.1). A state of chronic inflammation is a common feature of frailty syndrome. Thus, frailty can be considered as a clinical manifestation of cardiovascular disease, where senescence may be the connection. Significant advances in our understanding of cellular senescence and the proof of concept that interventions able to modulate the fundamental mechanisms of aging, may significantly impact on health as well as

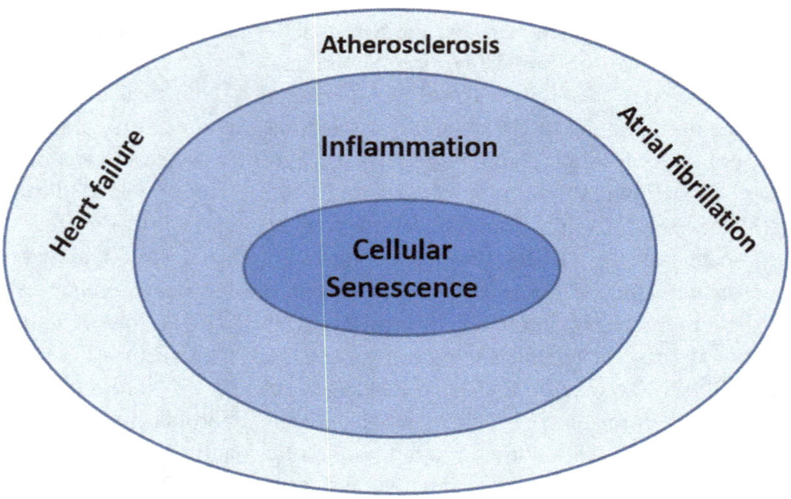

Fig. 9.1 Conceptual framework. The cellular senescence linked to inflammation and cardiovascular diseases

morbidities compression. Some strategic approaches are trying to protect against cardiomyocyte loss and thus to improve myocardial structure and performance, as well. The prevention of senescent cells accumulation in cardiac tissue or their cleaning, in the right amount, may delay the onset of CVDs. In progeroid mice (Xu et al. 2015) it has been shown that senolytics—the class of small molecules under basic research able to induce death of senescent cells—are effective in reducing frailty. However, the toxicity of these drugs remains a major concern and limitation in human studies.

References

Acosta JC, Banito A, Wuestefeld T, Georgilis A, Janich P, Morton JP, Athineos D, Kang TW, Lasitschka F, Andrulis M, Pascual G, Morris KJ, Khan S, Jin H, Dharmalingam G, Snijders AP, Carroll T, Capper D, Pritchard C, Inman GJ, Longerich T, Sansom OJ, Benitah SA, Zender L, Gil J (2013) A complex secretory program orchestrated by the inflammasome controls paracrine senescence. Nat Cell Biol 15 (8):978–990. https://doi.org/10.1038/ncb2784

Afilalo J, Alexander KP, Mack MJ et al (2014) Frailty assessment in the cardiovascular care of older adults. J Am Coll Cardiol 63:747–762. https://doi.org/10.1016/j.jacc.2013.09.070

Afilalo J, Karunananthan S, Eisenberg MJ et al (2009) Role of frailty in patients with cardiovascular disease. Am J Cardiol 103:1616–1621. https://doi.org/10.1016/j.amjcard.2009.01.375

Boccardi V, Comanducci C, Baroni M, Mecocci P (2017) Of energy and entropy: the ineluctable impact of aging in old age dementia. Int J Mol Sci 18(12). pii:E2672. https://doi.org/10.3390/ijms18122672

Centurione L, Antonucci A, Miscia S et al (2002) Age-related death-survival balance in myocardium: an immunohistochemical and biochemical study. Mech Ageing Dev 123:341–350

Cesari M, Penninx BWJH, Pahor M et al (2004) Inflammatory markers and physical performance in older persons: the InCHIANTI study. J Gerontol A Biol Sci Med Sci 59:242–248

Collard RM, Boter H, Schoevers RA, Oude Voshaar RC (2012) Prevalence of Frailty in community-dwelling older persons: a systematic review. J Am Geriatr Soc 60:1487–1492. https://doi.org/10.1111/j.1532-5415.2012.04054.x

Dantzer R (2009) Cytokine, sickness behavior, and depression. Immunol Allergy Clin North Am 29:247–264. https://doi.org/10.1016/j.iac.2009.02.002

DeMello M, Ross SA, Briel M et al (2015) Association between shortened leukocyte telomere length and cardiometabolic outcomes: systematic review and meta-analysis. Circ Cardiovasc Genet 8:4–7. https://doi.org/10.1161/CIRCGENETICS.113.000485

Dumurgier J, Elbaz A, Ducimetière P et al (2009) Slow walking speed and cardiovascular death in well functioning older adults: prospective cohort study. BMJ 339:b4460. https://doi.org/10.1136/bmj.b4460

Ferrucci L, Levine ME, Kuo PL, Simonsick EM (2018) Time and the metrics of aging. Circ Res 123(7):740–744

Fried LP, Ferrucci L, Darer J et al (2004) Untangling the concepts of disability, frailty, and comorbidity: implications for improved targeting and care. J Gerontol A Biol Sci Med Sci 59:255–263

Hayflick L, Moorhead PS (1961) The serial cultivation of human diploid cell strains. Exp Cell Res 25:585–621

Katsuumi G, Shimizu I, Yoshida Y, Minamino T (2018) Vascular senescence in cardiovascular and metabolic diseases. Front Cardiovasc Med 5:18. https://doi.org/10.3389/fcvm.2018.00018

Kawashima S, Yokoyama M (2004) Dysfunction of endothelial nitric oxide synthase and atherosclerosis. Arterioscler Thromb Vasc Biol 24:998–1005. https://doi.org/10.1161/01.ATV.0000125114.88079.96

Kortlever RM, Higgins PJ, Bernards R (2006) Plasminogen activator inhibitor-1 is a critical downstream target of p53 in the induction of replicative senescence. Nat Cell Biol 8:877–884. https://doi.org/10.1038/ncb1448

Kotecha D, Piccini JP (2015) Atrial fibrillation in heart failure: what should we do? Eur Heart J 36:ehv513. https://doi.org/10.1093/eurheartj/ehv513

Krouwer VJD, Hekking LHP, Langelaar-Makkinje M et al (2012) Endothelial cell senescence is associated with disrupted cell-cell junctions and increased monolayer permeability. Vasc Cell 4:12. https://doi.org/10.1186/2045-824X-4-12

Lakatta EG, Levy D (2003) Arterial and cardiac aging: major shareholders in cardiovascular disease enterprises: Part II: the aging heart in health: links to heart disease. Circulation 107:346–354

Lee WJ, Chen LK, Liang CK et al (2016) Soluble ICAM-1, independent of IL-6, is associated with prevalent frailty in community-dwelling elderly Taiwanese people. PLoS ONE 11:e0157877. https://doi.org/10.1371/journal.pone.0157877

Leng SX, Tian X, Matteini A et al (2011) Il-6-independent association of elevated serum neopterin levels with prevalent frailty in community-dwelling older adults. Age Ageing 40:475–481. https://doi.org/10.1093/ageing/afr047

Leng SX, Xue Q-L, Tian J et al (2009) Associations of neutrophil and monocyte counts with frailty in community-dwelling disabled older women: results from the women's health and aging studies I. Exp Gerontol 44:511–516. https://doi.org/10.1016/j.exger.2009.05.005

Leri A, Franco S, Zacheo A et al (2003) Ablation of telomerase and telomere loss leads to cardiac dilatation and heart failure associated with p53 upregulation. EMBO J 22:131–139. https://doi.org/10.1093/emboj/cdg013

López-Otín C, Blasco MA, Partridge L et al (2013) The hallmarks of aging. Cell 153:1194–1217. https://doi.org/10.1016/j.cell.2013.05.039

Matsuzawa Y, Konishi M, Akiyama E et al (2013) Association between gait speed as a measure of frailty and risk of cardiovascular events after myocardial infarction. J Am Coll Cardiol 61:1964–1972. https://doi.org/10.1016/j.jacc.2013.02.020

Matthews C, Gorenne I, Scott S et al (2006) Vascular smooth muscle cells undergo telomere-based senescence in human atherosclerosis: effects of telomerase and oxidative stress. Circ Res 99:156–164. https://doi.org/10.1161/01.RES.0000233315.38086.bc

Meyer K, Hodwin B, Ramanujam D et al (2016) Essential Role for premature senescence of myofibroblasts in myocardial fibrosis. j am coll cardiol 67:2018–2028. https://doi.org/10.1016/j.jacc.2016.02.047

Minamino T, Komuro I (2002) Role of telomere in endothelial dysfunction in atherosclerosis. Curr Opin Lipidol 13:537–543

Nadruz W, Kitzman D, Windham BG et al (2017) Cardiovascular dysfunction and frailty among older adults in the community: the ARIC study. J Gerontol A Biol Sci Med Sci 72:958–964. https://doi.org/10.1093/gerona/glw199

Newman AB, Gottdiener JS, Mcburnie MA et al (2001) Associations of subclinical cardiovascular disease with frailty. J Gerontol A Biol Sci Med Sci 56:M158–M166

Quijano C, Cao L, Fergusson MM et al (2012) Oncogene-induced senescence results in marked metabolic and bioenergetic alterations. Cell Cycle 11:1383–1392. https://doi.org/10.4161/cc.19800

Rippe C, Blimline M, Magerko KA et al (2012) MicroRNA changes in human arterial endothelial cells with senescence: relation to apoptosis, eNOS and inflammation. Exp Gerontol 47:45–51. https://doi.org/10.1016/j.exger.2011.10.004

Scherbov S, Weber D (2017) Future trends in the prevalence of severe activity limitations among older adults in Europe: a cross-national population study using EU-SILC. BMJ Open 7:e017654. https://doi.org/10.1136/bmjopen-2017-017654

Soysal P, Stubbs B, Lucato P et al (2016) Inflammation and frailty in the elderly: a systematic review and meta-analysis. Ageing Res Rev 31:1–8. https://doi.org/10.1016/j.arr.2016.08.006

van Deursen JM (2014) The role of senescent cells in ageing. Nature 509:439–446. https://doi.org/10.1038/nature13193

Wang JC, Bennett M (2012) Aging and atherosclerosis: mechanisms, functional consequences, and potential therapeutics for cellular senescence. Circ Res 111:245–259. https://doi.org/10.1161/CIRCRESAHA.111.261388

Xu M, Tchkonia T, Ding H et al (2015) JAK inhibition alleviates the cellular senescence-associated secretory phenotype and frailty in old age. Proc Natl Acad Sci U S A 112:E6301–E6310. https://doi.org/10.1073/pnas.1515386112

Yoshida Y, Shimizu I, Katsuumi G et al (2015) p53-Induced inflammation exacerbates cardiac dysfunction during pressure overload. J Mol Cell Cardiol 85:183–198. https://doi.org/10.1016/j.yjmcc.2015.06.001

Zhang J, Patel JM, Block ER (2002) Enhanced apoptosis in prolonged cultures of senescent porcine pulmonary artery endothelial cells. Mech Ageing Dev 123:613–625

Comprehensive Geriatric Assessment in Cardiovascular Disease

10

Jacopo Demurtas, Fiona Ecarnot, Simone Cernesi, Marco Solari, Miguel Angel Munoz and Alberto Cella

Abstract

Frailty and cardiovascular disease (CVD) are both highly prevalent in older adults. Cardiovascular disease has been identified as the most frequent cause of death, while frailty has been identified as one of geriatric giants characterized by decreased physiological reserves and increased vulnerability. However, the exact pathobiological links between the two conditions have not been fully elucidated. Consequently, we observe a relevant difficulty not only in accurately defining cardiovascular risk in vulnerable elderly patients (and the other way around), but also a lack of consensus regarding CVD management in the very old. Nowadays, considering the enormous technical innovation, many elderly patients, if appropriately selected, could be eligible even for the most complex treatments, including invasive cardiological procedures. Identification of frail patients at risk of negative outcomes can allow the customization of therapeutic interventions in elderly patients with CVD, allowing the elderly who can benefit from them to undergo even invasive procedures and avoiding futile or dangerous treatments for the most vulnerable patients. A large number of tools and definitions for assessing frailty have been proposed; different scales and assessment tools can be useful for different purposes, but at present there is no clear indication for their use in CVD. In this chapter, we will describe the main geriatric approach to ascertain frailty, the assessment tools used in patients with cardiovascular

J. Demurtas (✉)
Primary Care Department, Azienda USL Toscana Sud Est, AFT Orbetello, Grosseto, Italy
e-mail: eritrox7@gmail.com

F. Ecarnot
Department of Cardiology, University Hospital Jean Minjoz, and EA3920, University of Franche-Comté, 25000 Besançon, France

S. Cernesi
Azienda USL Modena, Modena, Italy

M. Solari
Cardiology Unit, Ospedale Misericordia, Azienda USL Toscana Sud Est, Grosseto, Italy

M. A. Munoz
Primary Care Research Unit IDIAP-Jordi Gol, Barcelona, Spain

M. A. Munoz
Departament de Salut, Institut Català de la Salut, IDIAP-Jordi Gol, Generalitat de Catalunya, Barcelona, Spain

M. A. Munoz
School of Medicine, Universitat Autònoma de Barcelona, Barcelona, Spain

M. A. Munoz
European General Practice Research Network, European Primary Care Cardiovascular Society, Barcelona, Spain

A. Cella
Intermediate Care Unit (Department of Geriatric Care, OrthoGeriatrics and Rehabilitation), E.O. Galliera Hospital, Genoa, Italy

N. Veronese (ed.), *Frailty and Cardiovascular Diseases*, Advances in Experimental Medicine and Biology 1216, https://doi.org/10.1007/978-3-030-33330-0_10

diseases, and propose an operational strategy to evaluate frailty and identify patients eligible for pharmacologic or surgical interventions.

Keywords
Frailty assessment · Risk stratification · Cardiovascular diseases · Heart failure · Transcatheter aortic valve replacement · TAVR

10.1 Introduction

In older adults, both cardiovascular disease (CVD) and frailty are highly prevalent and often coexist (Stewart 2019; Veronese et al. 2017). Cardiovascular diseases still represent the main cause of morbidity and mortality among older adults. In the European Union, almost 49 million individuals have CVD, and there are approximately 4.1 million deaths from CVD each year, of which over 80% occur in persons aged 65 years and over (Singh et al. 2014). The burden of CVD disproportionately affects older people, in whom overall health status, particularly frailty, is known to influence prognosis (Singh et al. 2014). Frailty is a state of multi-system impairment leading to decreased physiological reserve and increased vulnerability to stressors (Clegg et al. 2013). There is a bidirectional relationship between CVD and frailty, with many common pathways and risk factors being implicated in both conditions (Stewart 2019). Patients with CVD are more likely to become frail (Kleipool et al. 2018), while the presence of frailty is associated with several pathological conditions across the spectrum of CVD, including heart failure (McNallan et al. 2013; Volpato et al. 2011), cardiac surgery (Lee et al. 2010; Sundermann et al. 2011), atrial fibrillation (Polidoro et al. 2013; Perera et al. 2009; Lefebvre et al. 2016), severe valvular heart disease (Green et al. 2012; Schoenenberger et al. 2013; Stortecky et al. 2012; Ewe et al. 2010), and coronary artery disease (Ekerstad et al. 2011; Purser et al. 2006; Singh et al. 2011; White et al. 2016). Older patients with CVD are often affected by multimorbidity and frailty—which in turn affect clinical manifestations, prognosis, and response to treatment—and are associated with inflammation by mechanisms similar to those in CVD. The hypothesis that inflammation affects CVD, multimorbidity, and frailty by inhibiting growth factors, increasing catabolism, and interfering with homeostatic signalling is attractive but requires confirmation in humans (19bis). Nowadays, thanks to advances in technical innovations, large numbers of older patients, previously considered ineligible for the most complex cardiological therapies, are now be treated with devices, procedures and pharmacological therapies that were heretofore reserved for younger patients (Dodson and Maurer 2011). These novel and advanced cardiovascular therapeutic treatments have contributed to increase the overall life expectancy and led to an increasing number of older adults living with chronic CVD-, this represents an enormous clinical and socio-economic burden for Western society (Kleipool et al. 2018).

Identifying persons at high risk of frailty among this growing population of older adults may enable earlier implementation of interventions targeted to those most likely to benefit (Stewart 2019), and help to counteract the symbiotic effect of the combined presence of frailty and CVD.

In this context, the issue of appropriate patient assessment has become crucial in clinical practice. Indeed, on the one hand, there is a need to avoid under-treatment of older adults based simply on their chronological age, while on the other hand, it is increasingly important to optimize resource allocation to prevent patients from receiving futile and costly interventions (Afilalo et al. 2014). The majority of standardized scores for risk stratification in CVD have been developed and validated in middle-aged adults. However, in the elderly population the value of existing risk scores in discriminating between potential benefit and harm from a specific management strategy or intervention is currently unreliable. Moreover, since frail older people are often excluded from clinical trials, standardized guidelines are often not useful in the very old adult with significant multi-morbidity, polypharmacy, and in whom goals of care should be focused less on mortality and more on quality of life and maintaining independence (Bell and Saraf 2014). Indeed, existing risk stratification tools do not take into account variables that reflect frailty status, even though frailty is known to be associated with a twofold increase in mortality risk in CVD (Afilalo et al. 2014). Hence, there is a compelling need for assessment tools that account for the complexity of older individuals, and are able to measure the multiple determinants of frailty and stratify risk due not only to the severity of CVD itself, but also to the overall functional status of the older person. The recognition of frail older subjects may enable better estimates of prognosis, and consequently, avoidance of potentially useless, time- and cost-consuming medical interventions in these patients (Gill 2012).

10.2 Screening and Diagnosis of Frailty in Elderly People

The Royal College of Physicians and the French Society of Geriatrics and Gerontology advocated screening for frailty in older persons. Simple rapid screening tests have been developed and validated to allow physicians to rapidly recognize frail persons (Morley et al. 2013): examples of some commonly used screening tools include the FRAIL scale (Morley et al. 2012), the Gérontopôle Frailty Screening Tool (Subra et al. 2012) and the Edmonton Frail Scale (Rolfson et al. 2006). This latter scale is a simpler tool that does not require special training; it includes short questions about multiple domains, such as cognition assessed by the clock drawing test, self-reported general health, functional independence, social support, medication use, mood, continence, and functional performance.

Recent reviews, however, highlight that only few frailty screening measures seem to be valid, reliable and accurate, and with good predictive ability. Among them, the Frailty Index, Prisma-7 (Turner and Clegg 2014) and some physical performance tests emerged as the most useful in routine care and community settings (Apóstolo et al. 2017; Clegg et al. 2014).

Indeed, several studies have reported that single indicators of functional capacity such as grip strength (Celis-Morales et al. 2018), walk speed (Studenski et al. 2011; Hardy et al. 2007) and the "timed up and go test (TUG)" (Bischoff et al. 2003) are good predictors of adverse outcomes.

One of the most widely used performance test is the Short Physical Performance Battery (SPPB), which includes three tests exploring balance, gait, and, indirectly, via repeated chair standing, lower limb strength (Guralnik et al. 1994). Population-based cohort studies (Di Bari et al. 2006) have demonstrated that the SPPB is a strong, independent predictor of mortality, institutionalization, and incident disability in old age. In subjects older than 65 years living in the community, the risk of death and disability increased 7–9% for every point reduction in SPPB score, even after adjustment for complex measures of comorbidity (Di Bari et al. 2006). In patients hospitalized for an acute medical event, in most cases congestive heart failure (HF), SPBB is a powerful short- and long-term predictor of overall clinical and functional status, length of hospital stay, rehospitalization, or death (Volpato et al. 2011).

Another widely used measure of physical performance is gait speed, which has been proposed as a novel "vital sign" for older persons. It has been shown to be a good predictor of survival and other hard endpoints in older populations (Hardy et al. 2007; Bischoff et al. 2003). Gait speed is usually evaluated over a short distance (4 or 5 m), walking at a usual, comfortable speed. Accepted cutoffs vary between 0.8 and 1 m/s, depending on the purpose of the examination.

We must also give an account of the recent lively debate between two 'schools of thought' about the two instruments that represent the most known operational definitions of frailty, i.e. the frailty phenotype (proposed and validated by Fried and colleagues in the Cardiovascular Health Study) (Fried et al. 2001) and the Frailty Index (FI) (proposed and validated by Rockwood and colleagues in the Canadian Study of Health and Aging) (Rockwood and Mitnitski 2012). The two instruments have different purposes but can be complementary in the evaluation of the older person: the frailty phenotype may be more suitable for an immediate identification of non-disabled elders at risk of negative events, while the FI may summarize the results of a comprehensive geriatric assessment providing a marker of deficits accumulation (Cesari et al. 2013). Linda Fried et al. proposed a definition of frailty mainly based on physical performance parameters. They proposed 5 clinical criteria, namely weakness assessed from grip strength, slow walk speed, self-reported exhaustion, low physical activity, and unintentional weight loss. The Fried criteria for frailty are met when 3 or more of these 5 characteristics are present (Fried et al. 2001).

The 'original' version of the FI was composed by a long checklist of clinical conditions and diseases (70 items); it has been reported that estimates of risk are robust when a minimum of 50 items are considered, but shorter versions (as low as 20 conditions) have also been explored. The conceptual design of this index deems as more important the deficit accumulation. The 7-point CSHA Clinical Frailty Scale (Rockwood et al. 2005) grades frailty on a broad assessment of functional capacity and general health from "very fit," robust, energetic, well nourished, motivated, and fit, to "very severely frail," i.e. completely dependent on others for the activities of daily living or terminal. When evaluated by geriatricians, frailty is a strong predictor of both mortality and need for institutional care (Rockwood et al. 2005). However, this scale is relatively subjective, influencing consistency of assessment between clinicians.

Frailty assessment by evaluating accumulated clinical deficits has been extended to the Electronic Frailty Index, which can automatically calculate a frailty score with data from electronic medical records (Clegg et al. 2016).

The "hospital frailty risk score" (Gilbert et al. 2018) assesses the risk of frailty from algorithms using multiple ICD-10 codes. However, frailty based on ICD-10 codes showed only fair to moderate agreement with clinical measures of frailty (Gilbert et al. 2018).

However, to date only the Comprehensive Geriatric Assessment (CGA) is considered the gold standard for the diagnosis of frailty in elderly patients (Turner and Clegg 2014). CGA is a multidisciplinary and multidimensional process aimed at capturing information on accumulated clinical and functional deficits, nutrition, social factors, and cognitive function (Ellis et al. 2017); consequently, this evaluation can be very informative regarding the specific factors contributing to frailty. CGA has not only a diagnostic purpose but has also proved to be an effective management tool for the health needs of the elderly in several health conditions and in different clinical contexts (Pilotto et al. 2017). CGA however requires time and specialized geriatric skills, so it cannot be applied to all the elderly but only to those who can benefit the most, namely those not too fit and those not too clinically compromised or with reduced life expectancy (Rubenstein 1995).

Aggregated multidimensional indices (like FI by Rockwood) are able to combine feasibility and typical information content of the CGA in a 'summary' form, overcoming the methodological complexity of the CGA.

The Multidimensional Prognostic Index (MPI) is another aggregate index based on a standardized CGA that was developed and validated for 1-month and 1-year mortality in two large cohorts of hospitalized patients aged over 65 years (Pilotto et al. 2008). The MPI has been used and validated in numerous cohorts of elderly patients suffering from specific acute and chronic pathologies, always showing excellent clinimetric properties in stratifying elderly subjects in different risk groups both for short and long term mortality, as confirmed by reliable systematic reviews (Yourman et al. 2012; Dent et al. 2016).

10.3 Frailty Assessment in CVD

Among patients with CVD, frailty is up to three times more common (von Haehling et al. 2013), and reportedly affects over 40% of those aged over 70 years of age admitted to a cardiology unit with acute CVD (Sanchez et al. 2011) and about half of elderly patients with heart failure (Denfeld et al. 2017).

Although there is increasing awareness of the importance of frailty in adjusting risk assessment in patients with CVD, there is no consensus as to the best tool to be used for the evaluation of frailty in this clinical context given that no validated frailty instruments specific to heart failure (HF) or other cardiovascular conditions are available (Forman and Alexander 2016; McDonagh et al. 2018).

A recent systematic review (McDonagh et al. 2018) identified seven frailty assessment instruments that have been used in HF research heretofore, namely the Frailty Phenotype, the Deficit Accumulation Index, the Tilburg Frailty Indicator, the CGA, the Frailty Staging System, the Canadian Health and Ageing Clinical Frailty Scale and the Survey of Health, Ageing and Retirement in Europe Frailty Index. Among these, none has been validated for use in HF, although assessing frailty with a validated instrument is a priority, as recommended by international frailty guidelines (Morley et al. 2013; Dent et al. 2017).

In any case, however, some frailty measures have proved to be able to stratify the risk of negative clinical events in different cardiological conditions and in the context of invasive cardiological procedures or even cardiac surgery.

A systematic review and meta-analysis about frailty and mortality after percutaneous coronary intervention (PCI) showed that frailty (measured by means of Fried score or CSHA) was a significant predictor of all-cause mortality after the procedure, with a mean hazard ratio (HR) of about 3 (Tse et al. 2017).

The role of MPI as a prognostic tool for 30-day mortality has also been tested even in older adults discharged after hospitalization for HF (Pilotto et al. 2010). In this cohort of 376 patients aged over 65 admitted to a geriatric unit with a diagnosis of HF, increasing MPI grades were associated with progressively higher 30-day mortality rates in both men and women.

The discriminatory capacity of MPI was also good, with an area under the ROC curve for mortality of 0.83 (95% CI, 0.76–0.90) in men and of 0.80 (95% CI, 0.71–0.89) in women. In the same study, MPI was compared with other "traditional" prognostic scores, and the predictive value of MPI was found to be higher than that of the New York Heart Association (NYHA), the Enhanced Feedback for Effective Cardiac Treatment (EFFECT), and the Acute Decompensated Heart Failure National Registry (ADHERE) models in both men and in women (Pilotto et al. 2010). A sensitive measure of multidimensional impairment such as the MPI could be useful in identifying older CVD patients with a different risk of mortality, who could then be oriented to the most appropriate management depending on their individual circumstances.

In the frame of the MPI_AGE project (Bureau et al. 2017), a prospective observational study was carried out in consecutive patients aged ≥ 75 years who underwent transcatheter aortic valve implantation (TAVI) . MPI was calculated at baseline and after 1-year of follow-up. Among 116 patients (mean age 86.2 $\pm$ 4.2 years, mean MPI score 0.39 $\pm$ 0.13), the mortality rate was higher for higher MPI scores at 6 and 12 months. Patient survival also decreased in line with increasing MPI scores (HR = 2.83, 95% CI 1.38–5.82, $p = 0.004$). This study indicates that CGA-based MPI was an accurate tool to predict prognosis and contribute to selection of older patients suitable for the TAVI procedure (Bureau et al. 2017).

Another study, the CGA-TAVI, focused on gathering data on CGA results and medium-term outcomes in geriatric patients undergoing TAVI (Ungar et al. 2018). In a total of 71 patients undergoing TAVI, the authors reported that after adjustment for selected baseline characteristics, a higher MPI score and a lower SPPB score were significantly associated with an increased likelihood of death and/or hospitalisation in the first 3 months after the procedure. The use of CGA during clinical assessment of the operative risk in patients with aortic stenosis (AS) has been suggested as a way to address the shortcomings of the EuroSCORE and STS score, and to better predict outcomes (Ekerstad et al. 2011; Guralnik et al. 1994). Interestingly, in the study by Ungar et al. (2018), while high MPI was a "negative predictor" in the univariate analysis, it became a "positive predictor" after adjusting for age, gender, NYHA class and surgical risk. This change of direction can be explained by the clinical setting; younger patients with a low MPI are typically treated with surgical aortic valve replacement (SAVR), while older patients with a high MPI are unlikely to be treated at all. Consequently, the reported TAVI population was likely composed of patients with a lower age and high MPI or a higher age and low MPI, resulting in a switch of the direction of the odds ratio by multivariate analysis. This reflection of the clinical context is supportive of the "real" association between MPI score and outcomes (Ungar et al. 2018).

Although no other studies appear to have specifically reported on the predictive value of MPI in TAVI, several studies (Pilotto et al. 2009, 2010; Giantin et al. 2013; Sancarlo et al. 2012) have shown higher MPI scores to be significantly associated with higher mortality in older patients with a variety of acute illnesses, including HF and transient ischemic attack (TIA).

Other studies have evaluated multi-component models for predicting mortality and morbidity after cardiac invasive procedures. For TAVI specifically, Green et al. found that patients with a high frailty score, as determined by gait speed, grip strength, serum albumin and activities of daily living (ADL), were at greater risk of one-year mortality (Green et al. 2012). The five-component frailty score proposed by Kamga et al. was able to predict one-year mortality after transfemoral TAVI (Kamga et al. 2013). Stortecky et al. (2012) identified numerous parameters in their Multidimensional Geriatric Assessment that were predictive of 30-day and one-year mortality and major adverse cardiovascular and cerebral events (MACCE) after TAVI. Data from the PARTNER trial (Arnold et al. 2014) were used to construct models for predicting a poor outcome, defined as death or a low/significantly decreased quality of life, after TAVI (Arnold et al. 2016). These models were subsequently validated in a large multi-centre cohort of TAVI patients, with an incremental increase in discriminatory capacity with the addition of markers of frailty and disability (Arnold et al. 2016). In agreement with the data from the CGA registry (Ungar et al. 2018), these studies demonstrate the potential value of such multicomponent analyses for predicting outcome after TAVI. In the same work, it was reported that use of the SPPB alone was equally as effective as the MPI for predicting death and/or hospitalisation, and death and/or non-fatal stroke, in the first 3 months after TAVI (Ungar et al. 2018). This short series of tests is recommended by the European Union Geriatric Medicine Society (EuGMS) as part of CGA in older people (Ekerstad et al. 2011), although it appears that there is little published evidence in support of its use for assessing TAVI candidates specifically. The concept of tests of physical ability to predict outcome after TAVI or cardiac surgery has been evaluated in other studies. Stortecky et al. reported that the "timed get-up and go" (TUG) test had the greatest predictive ability of all the individual geriatric assessment tools that they investigated (Schoenenberger et al. 2013). In combination with either the STS or EuroSCORE, the TUG was superior to the other components evaluated for predicting all-cause mortality and MACCE during the first year after TAVI. A recent report by the American College of Cardiology (ACC) recommends that a 5 m gait speed test and a 6 min walk test be used to assess frailty and physical functioning, respectively, when determining a patient's suitability for TAVI.

The simplicity of physical tests such as gait speed and SPPB is not their only one advantage. The lack of subjectivity on the part of both physician and patient provides a level of accuracy that cannot be obtained using questionnaire-based assessment. This is particularly relevant for the advanced-age cardiologic population, where cognitive impairment is a potentially significant confounding factor when evaluating self-reported parameters (Ioannidis 2009). The only limitation to the use of physical performance tests to stratify frailty in CVD is the possible presence of physical disability not related to frailty.

SPPB has been applied to older patients being discharged from hospital after an episode of worsening HF, and was shown to accurately predict 1-year survival independently of demographics, comorbidity and regardless of ejection fraction and New York Heart Association classification, both of which are recognized as cornerstones of risk stratification in heart failure patients (Chiarantini et al. 2010).

Still in the context of the use of physical performance tests in CVD, it is worth mentioning some relevant data regarding the predictive role of gait speed. A meta-analysis of 44 articles totaling over 100,000 participants found that after adjustment for a median of 9 confounders, each reduction of 0.1 m/s in gait speed was associated with a 12% increase in the risk of early mortality and a significant 8% increase in the risk of CVD (Veronese et al. 2018). Furthermore, gait speed has been shown to improve risk stratification for adverse outcomes after cardiac surgery, percutaneous coronary intervention, and transcatheter aortic valve implantation (Afilalo et al. 2014; Afilalo et al. 2017). In particular, when assessing surgical risk for surgical aortic valve replacement, frailty evaluation was shown to increase the prognostic value of the traditional, validated score, namely the Society of Thoracic Surgeons (STS) risk score, in the Frailty ABCs (Frailty Assessment Before Cardiac Surgery) prospective study (Afilalo et al. 2010). In this study, Afilalo et al. reported that for a given STS risk prediction for mortality or major morbidity, the predicted risk based on the model including gait speed was 2–3 times greater in patients with slow gait compared to patients with normal gait speed (Afilalo et al. 2010).

Finally, a brief comment on the Essential Frailty Toolset (EFT) (Afilalo et al. 2017), a particular multi-dimensional tool used for assessing the potential for functional recovery in older adults undergoing transcatheter aortic valve replacement (TAVR) or surgical aortic valve replacement (SAVR). It includes physical function, assessed by chair rises, cognitive function, low serum albumin (<3.5 g/dL), and low hemoglobin (<13 g/dL in men, <12 g/dL in women). Compared to other frailty measures, EFT showed similar or better predictive ability for mortality and hospitalization, probably because in addition to assessment of physical and cognitive function, it includes measures of hepatic protein synthesis and hemopoiesis, which are powerful mortality predictors not included in most frailty scores (Afilalo et al. 2017).

10.4 Operative Indications

The relevance of assessing frailty in patients with CVD is undeniable, to select older people who will benefit most from interventions with invasive therapeutic procedures. Given that health status is reduced in patients with HF and frailty, measuring patient-reported health status is pivotal for cardiovascular conditions, according to the American Heart Association (AHA) (Rumsfeld et al. 2013). Moreover, a position paper from the AHA, American College of Cardiology and American Geriatrics Society states that future guidelines should take into account the assessment of frailty domains as well as chronological age in the management of older patients with HF (Rich et al. 2016). As most older adults are not frail, however, chronological age is not a reliable indicator of biological age and health status. Frailty, for instance, has been found to be a better predictor of age-dependent heart rhythm disorders than age (Cho 2016).

Formal screening for frailty should be performed in every older patient who comes to medical attention for any reason, but in particular in the case of established diagnosis of CVD.

Based on the predictive ability demonstrated in many studies and given the characteristics of the tests, gait speed and SPPB can be a quick, easy and inexpensive way to identify cardiologic older patients who may be at increased risk of adverse outcomes.

If the presence of frailty or pre-frailty is suspected (SPPB <9 or gait speed <0.8 m/s), then CGA should be performed with appropriate tools. CGA-based tools such as the MPI that allow stratification of older patients facilitate clinical decision-making in terms of diagnostic and therapeutic choices. People at low risk of frailty, i.e., MPI-1, should be treated according to usual guidelines. Conversely, aged individuals at moderate or high risk of frailty (i.e., MPI-2 or MPI-3) should be managed with tailored interventions according to their frailty profile and prognosis. In this regard, considering early palliative care/supportive care, especially in MPI-3 category, is important not to say mandatory.

10.5 Concluding Remarks

Frailty and CVD are intricately linked in a bidirectional relationship relying on several common risk factors and pathways. Patients with CVD are at increased risk of becoming frail, while frailty is associated with a significant increase in the risk of adverse outcomes across the spectrum of CVD manifestations. In this regard, there is a large body of evidence supporting the utility of taking frailty into account when attempting to modify the risk of CVD in older patients, and particularly when assessing the risk-benefit ratio of specific therapeutic interventions in various forms of CVD. To date, there is no consensus regarding the optimal approach to assessing frailty in CVD, and a multitude of different tools exist, based either on the presence of core phenotypic domains, or on the cumulative deficits model. The choice of method will be influenced by the reasons for performing the assessment, the source of relevant information, and the time and skills of the assessor. Assessments based on information from medical records or ICD-10 codes can be applied to large populations, but their value for guiding individual patient care is uncertain. Frailty should not be systematically considered as a contra-indication to therapy, but rather as an additional factor to guide appropriate decision-making, in agreement with the patient's wishes and goals of care. Reaching a consensus on a validated tool (or tool set) would facilitate frailty assessment in CVD older patients in daily practice, and would enable comparison of results across studies. Future research might also focus on investigating whether addressing the components of frailty could have a positive impact on incident CVD or outcomes in patients with CVD, and conversely, whether frail CVD patients yield greater benefit from interventions and rehabilitation. As the number of frail patients (with and without CVD) looks set to increase substantially over the coming decades owing to the progressively population ageing, the clinical relevance of frailty assessment is undeniable, and routine assessment of frailty can improve the prognostic assessment and management of CVD older patients.

References

Afilalo J, Eisenberg MJ, Morin JF, Bergman H, Monette J, Noiseux N et al (2010) Gait speed as an incremental predictor of mortality and major morbidity in elderly patients undergoing cardiac surgery. J Am Coll Cardiol 56(20):1668–1676

Afilalo J, Alexander KP, Mack MJ, Maurer MS, Green P, Allen LA et al (2014) Frailty assessment in the cardiovascular care of older adults. J Am Coll Cardiol 63(8):747–762

Afilalo J, Lauck S, Kim DH, Lefevre T, Piazza N, Lachapelle K et al (2017) Frailty in Older adults undergoing aortic valve replacement: the FRAILTY-AVR study. J Am Coll Cardiol 70 (6):689–700

Apóstolo J, Cooke R, Bobrowicz-Campos E, Santana S, Marcucci M, Cano A et al (2017) Predicting risk and outcomes for frail older adults: an umbrella review of frailty screening tools. JBI Database Syst Rev Implement Rep 15(4):1154

Arnold SV, Reynolds MR, Lei Y, Magnuson EA, Kirtane AJ, Kodali SK et al (2014) Predictors of poor outcomes after transcatheter aortic valve replacement: results from the PARTNER (Placement of Aortic Transcatheter Valve) trial. Circulation 129(25):2682–2690

Arnold SV, Afilalo J, Spertus JA, Tang Y, Baron SJ, Jones PG et al (2016) Prediction of poor outcome after transcatheter aortic valve replacement. J Am Coll Cardiol 68(17):1868–1877

Bell SP, Saraf A (2014) Risk stratification in very old adults: how to best gauge risk as the basis of management choices for patients aged over 80. Prog Cardiovasc Dis 57(2):197–203

Bischoff HA, Stahelin HB, Monsch AU, Iversen MD, Weyh A, von Dechend M et al (2003) Identifying a cut-off point for normal mobility: a comparison of the timed 'up and go' test in community-dwelling and institutionalised elderly women. Age Ageing 32 (3):315–320

Bureau ML, Liuu E, Christiaens L, Pilotto A, Mergy J, Bellarbre F et al (2017) Using a multidimensional prognostic index (MPI) based on comprehensive geriatric assessment (CGA) to predict mortality in elderly undergoing transcatheter aortic valve implantation. Int J Cardiol 236:381–386

Celis-Morales CA, Welsh P, Lyall DM, Steell L, Petermann F, Anderson J et al (2018) Associations of grip strength with cardiovascular, respiratory, and cancer outcomes and all cause mortality: prospective cohort study of half a million UK Biobank participants. BMJ 361:k1651

Cesari M, Gambassi G, Abellan van Kan G, Vellas B (2013) The frailty phenotype and the frailty index: different instruments for different purposes. Age Ageing 43(1):10–12

Chiarantini D, Volpato S, Sioulis F, Bartalucci F, Del Bianco L, Mangani I et al (2010) Lower extremity performance measures predict long-term prognosis in older patients hospitalized for heart failure. J Card Fail. 16(5):390–395

Cho HC (2016) Age is just a number: frailty better evaluates age-dependent heart rhythm defects. J Physiol 594(23):6805

Clegg A, Young J, Iliffe S, Rikkert MO, Rockwood K (2013) Frailty in elderly people. Lancet (London, England). 381(9868):752–762

Clegg A, Rogers L, Young J (2014) Diagnostic test accuracy of simple instruments for identifying frailty in community-dwelling older people: a systematic review. Age Ageing 44(1):148–152

Clegg A, Bates C, Young J, Ryan R, Nichols L, Ann Teale E et al (2016) Development and validation of an electronic frailty index using routine primary care electronic health record data. Age Ageing 45(3):353–360

Denfeld QE, Winters-Stone K, Mudd JO, Gelow JM, Kurdi S, Lee CS (2017) The prevalence of frailty in heart failure: a systematic review and meta-analysis. Int J Cardiol 236:283–289

Dent E, Kowal P, Hoogendijk EO (2016) Frailty measurement in research and clinical practice: a review. Eur J Intern Med 31:3–10

Dent E, Lien C, Lim WS, Wong WC, Wong CH, Ng TP et al (2017) The Asia-Pacific clinical practice guidelines for the management of frailty. J Am Med Dir Assoc 18(7):564–575

Di Bari M, Virgillo A, Matteuzzi D, Inzitari M, Mazzaglia G, Pozzi C et al (2006) Predictive validity of measures of comorbidity in older community dwellers: the Insufficienza Cardiaca negli Anziani Residenti a Dicomano Study. J Am Geriatr Soc 54(2):210–216

Dodson JA, Maurer MS (2011) Changing nature of cardiac interventions in older adults. Aging Health 7 (2):283–295

Ekerstad N, Swahn E, Janzon M, Alfredsson J, Lofmark R, Lindenberger M et al (2011) Frailty is independently associated with short-term outcomes for elderly patients with non-ST-segment elevation myocardial infarction. Circulation 124(22):2397–2404

Ellis G, Gardner M, Tsiachristas A, Langhorne P, Burke O, Harwood RH et al (2017) Comprehensive geriatric assessment for older adults admitted to hospital. Cochrane Database Syst Rev 9:CD006211

Ewe SH, Ajmone Marsan N, Pepi M, Delgado V, Tamborini G, Muratori M et al (2010) Impact of left ventricular systolic function on clinical and echocardiographic outcomes following transcatheter aortic valve implantation for severe aortic stenosis. Am Heart J 160(6):1113–1120

Forman DE, Alexander KP (2016) Frailty: a vital sign for older adults with cardiovascular disease. Can J Cardiol 32(9):1082–1087

Fried LP, Tangen CM, Walston J, Newman AB, Hirsch C, Gottdiener J et al (2001a) Frailty in older adults: evidence for a phenotype. J Gerontol Ser A, Biol Sci Med Sci 56(3):M146–M156

Fried LP, Tangen CM, Walston J, Newman AB, Hirsch C, Gottdiener J et al (2001b) Frailty in older adults: evidence for a phenotype. J Gerontol A Biol Sci Med Sci 56(3):M146–M156

Giantin V, Valentini E, Iasevoli M, Falci C, Siviero P, De Luca E et al (2013) Does the Multidimensional Prognostic Index (MPI), based on a Comprehensive Geriatric Assessment (CGA), predict mortality in cancer patients? results of a prospective observational trial. J Geriatric Oncol 4(3):208–217

Gilbert T, Neuburger J, Kraindler J, Keeble E, Smith P, Ariti C et al (2018) Development and validation of a Hospital Frailty Risk Score focusing on older people in acute care settings using electronic hospital records: an observational study. Lancet 391(10132):1775–1782

Gill TM (2012) The central role of prognosis in clinical decision making. JAMA 307(2):199–200

Green P, Woglom AE, Genereux P, Daneault B, Paradis JM, Schnell S et al (2012) The impact of frailty status on survival after transcatheter aortic valve replacement in older adults with severe aortic stenosis: a single-center experience. JACC Cardiovasc Interv 5 (9):974–981

Guralnik JM, Simonsick EM, Ferrucci L, Glynn RJ, Berkman LF, Blazer DG et al (1994) A short physical performance battery assessing lower extremity function: association with self-reported disability and prediction of mortality and nursing home admission. J Gerontol 49(2):M85–M94

Hardy SE, Perera S, Roumani YF, Chandler JM, Studenski SA (2007) Improvement in usual gait speed predicts better survival in older adults. J Am Geriatr Soc 55(11):1727–1734

Ioannidis JP (2009) Integration of evidence from multiple meta-analyses: a primer on umbrella reviews, treatment networks and multiple treatments meta-analyses. CMAJ 181(8):488–493

Kamga M, Boland B, Cornette P, Beeckmans M, De Meester C, Chenu P et al (2013) Impact of frailty scores on outcome of octogenarian patients undergoing transcatheter aortic valve implantation. Acta Cardiol 68(6):599–606

Kleipool EE, Hoogendijk EO, Trappenburg MC, Handoko ML, Huisman M, Peters MJ et al (2018) Frailty in older adults with cardiovascular disease: cause, effect or both? Aging Dis 9(3):489–497

Lee DH, Buth KJ, Martin BJ, Yip AM, Hirsch GM (2010) Frail patients are at increased risk for mortality and prolonged institutional care after cardiac surgery. Circulation 121(8):973–978

Lefebvre MC, St-Onge M, Glazer-Cavanagh M, Bell L, Kha Nguyen JN, Viet-Quoc Nguyen P et al (2016) The effect of bleeding risk and frailty status on anticoagulation patterns in octogenarians with atrial fibrillation: the FRAIL-AF study. Can J Cardiol 32 (2):169–176

McDonagh J, Ferguson C, Newton PJ (2018a) Frailty assessment in heart failure: an overview of the multi-domain approach. Curr Heart Fail Rep 15 (1):17–23

McDonagh J, Martin L, Ferguson C, Jha SR, Macdonald PS, Davidson PM et al (2018b) Frailty assessment instruments in heart failure: a systematic review. Eur J Cardiovasc Nurs 17(1):23–35

McNallan SM, Singh M, Chamberlain AM, Kane RL, Dunlay SM, Redfield MM et al (2013) Frailty and healthcare utilization among patients with heart failure in the community. JACC Heart Fail 1(2):135–141

Morley JE, Malmstrom TK, Miller DK (2012) A simple frailty questionnaire (FRAIL) predicts outcomes in middle aged African Americans. J Nutr Health Aging 16(7):601–608

Morley JE, Vellas B, van Kan GA, Anker SD, Bauer JM, Bernabei R et al (2013) Frailty consensus: a call to action. J Am Med Dir Assoc 14(6):392–397

Perera V, Bajorek BV, Matthews S, Hilmer SN (2009) The impact of frailty on the utilisation of antithrombotic therapy in older patients with atrial fibrillation. Age Ageing 38(2):156–162

Pilotto A, Ferrucci L, Franceschi M, D'Ambrosio LP, Scarcelli C, Cascavilla L et al (2008) Development and validation of a multidimensional prognostic index for one-year mortality from comprehensive geriatric assessment in hospitalized older patients. Rejuvenation Res 11(1):151–161

Pilotto A, Addante F, Ferrucci L, Leandro G, D'Onofrio G, Corritore M et al (2009) The multidimensional prognostic index predicts short- and long-term mortality in hospitalized geriatric patients with pneumonia. J Gerontol Ser A, Biol Sci Med Sci 64(8):880–887

Pilotto A, Addante F, Franceschi M, Leandro G, Rengo G, D'Ambrosio P et al (2010) Multidimensional Prognostic Index based on a comprehensive geriatric assessment predicts short-term mortality in older patients with heart failure. Circ Heart Fail 3 (1):14–20

Pilotto A, Cella A, Pilotto A, Daragjati J, Veronese N, Musacchio C et al (2017) Three decades of comprehensive geriatric assessment: evidence coming from different healthcare settings and specific clinical conditions. J Am Med Dir Assoc 18(2):192 e1–192 e11

Polidoro A, Stefanelli F, Ciacciarelli M, Pacelli A, Di Sanzo D, Alessandri C (2013) Frailty in patients affected by atrial fibrillation. Arch Gerontol Geriatr 57 (3):325–327

Purser JL, Kuchibhatla MN, Fillenbaum GG, Harding T, Peterson ED, Alexander KP (2006) Identifying frailty in hospitalized older adults with significant coronary artery disease. J Am Geriatr Soc 54(11):1674–1681

Rich MW, Chyun DA, Skolnick AH, Alexander KP, Forman DE, Kitzman DW et al (2016) Knowledge gaps in cardiovascular care of the older adult population: a scientific statement from the American Heart Association, American College of Cardiology, and American Geriatrics Society. J Am Coll Cardiol 67 (20):2419–2440

Rockwood K, Mitnitski A (2012) How might deficit accumulation give rise to frailty. J Frailty Aging 1 (1):8–12

Rockwood K, Song X, MacKnight C, Bergman H, Hogan DB, McDowell I et al (2005) A global clinical measure of fitness and frailty in elderly people. CMAJ 173(5):489–495

Rolfson DB, Majumdar SR, Tsuyuki RT, Tahir A, Rockwood K (2006) Validity and reliability of the edmonton frail scale. Age Ageing 35(5):526–529

Rubenstein L (1995) An overview of comprehensive geriatric assessment: rationale, history, program models, basic components. Geriatric Assessment Technology, The State of the Art New York, NY. Springer

Rumsfeld JS, Alexander KP, Goff DC Jr, Graham MM, Ho PM, Masoudi FA et al (2013) Cardiovascular health: the importance of measuring patient-reported health status: a scientific statement from the American Heart Association. Circulation 127(22):2233–2249

Sancarlo D, Pilotto A, Panza F, Copetti M, Longo MG, D'Ambrosio P et al (2012) A Multidimensional Prognostic Index (MPI) based on a comprehensive geriatric assessment predicts short- and long-term all-cause mortality in older hospitalized patients with transient ischemic attack. J Neurol 259(4):670–678

Sanchez E, Vidan MT, Serra JA, Fernandez-Aviles F, Bueno H (2011) Prevalence of geriatric syndromes and impact on clinical and functional outcomes in older patients with acute cardiac diseases. Heart 97 (19):1602–1606

Schoenenberger AW, Stortecky S, Neumann S, Moser A, Juni P, Carrel T et al (2013) Predictors of functional decline in elderly patients undergoing transcatheter aortic valve implantation (TAVI). Eur Heart J 34 (9):684–692

Singh M, Rihal CS, Lennon RJ, Spertus JA, Nair KS, Roger VL (2011) Influence of frailty and health status on outcomes in patients with coronary disease undergoing percutaneous revascularization. Circ Cardiovasc Qual Outcomes 4(5):496–502

Singh M, Stewart R, White H (2014) Importance of frailty in patients with cardiovascular disease. Eur Heart J 35 (26):1726–1731

Stewart R (2019) Cardiovascular disease and frailty: what are the mechanistic links? Clin Chem 65(1):80–86

Stortecky S, Schoenenberger AW, Moser A, Kalesan B, Juni P, Carrel T et al (2012) Evaluation of multidimensional geriatric assessment as a predictor of mortality and cardiovascular events after transcatheter aortic valve implantation. JACC Cardiovasc Interv 5 (5):489–496

Studenski S, Perera S, Patel K, Rosano C, Faulkner K, Inzitari M et al (2011) Gait speed and survival in older adults. JAMA 305(1):50–58

Subra J, Gillette-Guyonnet S, Cesari M, Oustric S, Vellas B, Platform T (2012) The integration of frailty into clinical practice: preliminary results from the Gerontopole. J Nutr Health Aging 16(8):714–720

Sundermann S, Dademasch A, Rastan A, Praetorius J, Rodriguez H, Walther T, et al (2011) One-year follow-up of patients undergoing elective cardiac surgery assessed with the comprehensive assessment of frailty test and its simplified form. Interact Cardiovasc Thorac Surg 13(2):119–123 (discussion 23)

Tse G, Gong M, Nunez J, Sanchis J, Li G, Ali-Hasan-Al-Saegh S et al (2017) Frailty and mortality outcomes after percutaneous coronary intervention: a systematic review and meta-analysis. J Am Med Dir Assoc 18(12):1097. e1–1097.e10

Turner G, Clegg A (2014) Best practice guidelines for the management of frailty: a British Geriatrics Society, Age UK and Royal College of General Practitioners report. Age Ageing 43(6):744–747

Ungar A, Mannarino G, van der Velde N, Baan J, Thibodeau MP, Masson JB et al (2018) Comprehensive geriatric assessment in patients undergoing transcatheter aortic valve implantation—results from the CGA-TAVI multicentre registry. BMC Cardiovasc Disord 18(1):1

Veronese N, Cereda E, Stubbs B, Solmi M, Luchini C, Manzato E et al (2017) Risk of cardiovascular disease morbidity and mortality in frail and pre-frail older adults: results from a meta-analysis and exploratory meta-regression analysis. Ageing Res Rev 35:63–73

Veronese N, Stubbs B, Volpato S, Zuliani G, Maggi S, Cesari M et al (2018) Association between gait speed with mortality, cardiovascular disease and cancer: a systematic review and meta-analysis of prospective cohort studies. J Am Med Dir Assoc 19(11):981–988 e7

Volpato S, Cavalieri M, Sioulis F, Guerra G, Maraldi C, Zuliani G et al (2011) Predictive value of the short physical performance battery following hospitalization in older patients. J Gerontol A Biol Sci Med Sci 66 (1):89–96

von Haehling S, Anker SD, Doehner W, Morley JE, Vellas B (2013) Frailty and heart disease. Int J Cardiol 168(3):1745–1747

White HD, Westerhout CM, Alexander KP, Roe MT, Winters KJ, Cyr DD et al (2016) Frailty is associated with worse outcomes in non-ST-segment elevation acute coronary syndromes: Insights from the TaRgeted platelet Inhibition to cLarify the Optimal strateGy to medicallY manage Acute Coronary Syndromes (TRILOGY ACS) trial. Eur Heart J Acute Cardiovasc Care 5(3):231–242

Yourman LC, Lee SJ, Schonberg MA, Widera EW, Smith AK (2012) Prognostic indices for older adults: a systematic review. JAMA 307(2):182–192

Role of Frailty on Risk Stratification in Cardiac Surgery and Procedures

11

Samuele Baldasseroni, Alessandra Pratesi, Francesco Orso, Aldo Lo Forte, Anna Chiara Baroncini, Giulia Lucarelli, Camilla Ghiara, Francesca Caramelli, Niccolò Marchionni and Andrea Ungar

Abstract

The number of older people candidates for interventional cardiology, such as PCI but especially for transcatheter aortic valve implantation (TAVI) , would increase in the future. Generically, the surgical risk, the amount of complications in the perioperative period, mortality and severe disability remain significantly higher in the elderly than in younger. For this reason it's important to determine the indication for surgical intervention, using tools able to predict not only the classics outcome (length of stay, mortality), but also those more specifically geriatrics, correlate to frailty: delirium, cognitive deterioration, risk of institutionalization and decline in functional status. The majority of the most used surgical risks scores are often specialist-oriented and many variables are not considered. The need of a multidimensional diagnostic process, focused on detect frailty, in order to program a coordinated and integrated plan for treatment and long term follow up, led to the development of a specific geriatric tool: the Comprehensive Geriatric Assessment (CGA). The CGA has the aim to improve the prognostic ability of the current risk scores to capture short long term mortality and disability, and helping to resolve a crucial issue providing solid clinical indications to help physician in the definition of on interventional approach as futile. This tool will likely optimize the selection of TAVI older candidates could have the maximal benefit from the procedure.

Keywords

Frailty · Elderly · Geriatrics · Surgical risk scores · Cardiac surgery · TAVI · Comprehensive geriatric assessment · Disability

S. Baldasseroni · F. Orso · A. L. Forte · A. C. Baroncini · G. Lucarelli · C. Ghiara · F. Caramelli · A. Ungar (✉)
Geriatric Medicine Unit, University of Florence and Azienda Ospedaliero-Universitaria Careggi, Florence, Italy
e-mail: aungar@unifi.it

A. Pratesi
Internal Medicine Unit, San Giuseppe Hospital, Empoli, Italy

N. Marchionni
Cardiothoracovascular Department, University of Florence and Azienda Ospedaliero-Universitaria Careggi, Florence, Italy

A. Ungar
Hypertension Centre - Syncope Unit, University of Florence, Florence, Italy

11.1 The Complexity of Risk Assessment in Older Patients Candidate to Surgery

Over the past 20 years the number of older people undergoing surgery has been exponentially growing, with plans to reach in the US in

N. Veronese (ed.), *Frailty and Cardiovascular Diseases*, Advances in Experimental Medicine and Biology 1216, https://doi.org/10.1007/978-3-030-33330-0_11

the next few years more than 47% of the totality of the surgical activity (Etzioni et al. 2003), resulting in an increase in the percentage of elderly evaluated preoperatively for different surgical indications (Klopfenstein et al. 1998).

This phenomenon is due to the increase in the average length of life, the improvement of surgical and anesthetic techniques as well as a significant improvement in mortality and morbidity intra- and peri-operative (Goldstein et al. 2010; Kurian et al. 2010). Despite those improvements, risk of surgery, complications in the perioperative period, mortality and severe disability remain significantly higher in the elderly than in younger (Polanczyk et al. 2001).

The perioperative risk of surgery of a patient is one of the main factors determining the final indication for intervention. Although many surgical procedures can enhance the quality and duration of life, a careful assessment is able to decrease both predictable and untoward risk of adverse event for the patient, increasingly vulnerable and frail, and improve the outcome. This is even more true for the elderly, for which we need tools able to predict not only the classics outcome (such us length of stay, mortality), but also those more specifically geriatrics, such as delirium, cognitive deterioration, disability and risk of institutionalization.

A national survey in the United Kingdom identified some alert in pre operative assessment of co-morbidity, *frailty* and risk and a sub-optimal intra- and post-operative medical care in the cohort of elderly who died within 30 days of surgery (National Confidential Enquiry into Patient Outcome and Death 2010).

In international literature (Myles 2014) has been increasing interest in consider not only the evaluation of outcome measures typically included in clinical studies (survival, major complications, mitigation of symptoms), but also in the use of patient-centered outcomes and the use of disability-free survival as a primary outcome, which often represents the real major goal for elderly patients.

There are various factors to be considered in assessing the risk of surgery, generally divided into patient-related and surgery-specific risks (such as urgency and duration of the operation, type of surgery, possibility of bleeding). To date, in elective surgery the patient-related risk assessment often consists of an evaluation 1–4 weeks before intervention, consisting in complete a default medical record with medical history, physical exam, laboratory tests and radiological imaging. This information, usually collected by anaesthetist basing on ASA (American Society of Anesthesiologists) Physical Status Classification (American Society of Anesthesiologists. ASA Physical Status Classification System 2014), providing the possibility to organize further investigations before surgery, alerts support services and permits the option of admission on the day of surgery. This is could be considered sufficient for young or adult patients, but not for the older ones. Indeed, aging is associated with a paraphysiological or pathological decline of the functional reserve of multiple organ systems with reduced adaptation to stress, with an increasing prevalence of comorbidity and loss of functional autonomy often concomitant with a reduction in social resources.

Indeed, the aging process per se entails a progressive reduction of physical performance and overall autonomy. This process (Nakamura and Miyao 2007) in the first instance is, in its temporal trajectory, genetically determined, and is linked to the progressive modification of biological processes (Nakamura and Miyao 2007). Nevertheless its phenotype is individually influenced by the style and background, and by the history of diseases (Nakamura and Miyao 2007). For these reasons, a group of octogenarians is by definition not homogeneous. Chronological age is an independent risk factor for both surgical and anesthesia as demonstrated by an extensive literature: Naughton and Feneck (2007) showed in over 1500 patients with cardiovascular diseases that have an age >70 years increases the risk of death at 6 months 3.57 times (OR, 95% CI: 2.22–5.73) in elective non-cardiac surgery. The prognostic value of chronological age was later confirmed by the fact that it always be the first item of the biggest score of surgical risk score whether it be included as a continuous variable that dichotomous (Barnett and Moonesinghe

2011). Anyway, chronological age is not a factor excluding "per se" from the surgery whether elective or emergency.

Must be finally emphasized as some fundamental outcome for the evaluation of the operative risk in surgery are today still little considered in the scientific literature, such as the risk of prolonged stay in intensive care unit and of prolonged ventilation. The Society of Thoracic Surgeons established a Quality Measurement Task Force to develop a method to evaluate adult surgery quality of care (Shahian et al. 2007), within which there is "Postoperative Risk-Adjusted Major Morbidity", where a parameter of bad performance is occurrence of prolonged ventilation/intubation, as defined in STS website (The Society of Thoracic Surgeons 2006).

As it known, in elderly occurs many "para-physiological" and pathological change: a decline in pulmonary reserve and in renal function, an alteration of gastrointestinal physiology, *sarcopenia*. All these changes compromise the ability of older patients to tolerate surgical procedures and increase their risk of mortality and morbidity and of decline in functional status. It is clear that becoming familiar with method and tools able to detect these changes alone and as a whole is necessary to choose the right patient to candidate to surgery and to achieve better-tailored treatments when possible.

11.2 The Reliability and Validity of the Risk Scores in the Elderly

An accurate risk stratification of perioperative cardiac elderly patient should have different objectives; first, to identify those who can benefit of intervention and those who have a not sustainable operatory risk; second, to identify those who need intensive care in the postoperative period, preparing in advance an ICU. The ideal tool for risk stratification in the elderly waiting for surgery should be; reliable; usable, if possible, in elective surgery but also in emergency; tested and built for an elderly population, with information about the functional and cognitive status and the level of non-cardiac comorbidities that the geriatric literature has demonstrated to be able to predict prognosis (Barnett and Moonesinghe 2011).

To date, is privileged a purely anaesthetic, surgical or cardiological perspective in risk score. In fact, the score of surgical risk are often type specialist-oriented (anaesthetic or surgical or cardiology). One of the best-known risk score of the population is the 'American Society of Anesthesiologists Physical Status score ASA-PS) (Saklad 1941) (Table 11.1) which categorized patients in five types of populations at growing risk of anaesthesia, with a recently added ones dedicated to organ donors (American Society of Anesthesiologists 1963). As can be seen from Table 11.1 is easy to use and fast, but with several limitations: it is not adjusted for sex, age and anthropometric characteristics of patient, and is not applicable to geriatric patients not considering geriatric parameters. Recently, it has been demonstrated (Wolters et al. 1997) that the instrument has low individual predictive power, being capable to predict not more than 15–16% of perioperative complications, with a positive predictive power next to 50% and negative 80%, percentages to be considered really low (Wolters et al. 1997).

The most widely used surgical risk score is the POSSUM (The Physiological and Operative Severity Score for the enumeration of Mortality and Morbidity-POSSUM), developed in 1991 by Copeland et al. (1991). In its final version this score incorporates eighteen variables through two mathematical algorithms is constructed a risk value for mortality and morbidity (twelve physiological variables recorded before surgery and include symptoms, signs and laboratory test and six surgical variables). The POSSUM is used for the assessment of surgical procedures risk in both elective and emergency interventions for urology, vascular, hepatobiliary and gastrointestinal (Bennett-Guerrero et al. 2003). The POSSUM is reliable in predicting hospital mortality but has little power to seize the perioperative complications (Prytherch et al. 1998).

Regarding cardiac scores, an interesting risk score has been developed based on previous risk

Table 11.1 ASA grade

I A normal healthy patient
II A patient with mild systemic disease
III A patient with severe systemic disease
IV A patient with severe systemic disease that is a constant threat to life
V A moribund patient who is not expected to survive without the operation
VI A declared brain dead patient whose organs are being removed for donor purposes

Table 11.2 Revised Cardiac Risk Index-RCRI

1 *High-Risk Surgery*: Intraperitoneal; Intrathoracic; Suprainguinal vascular
2 *History of ischemic heart disease*: history of MI; history of positive exercise test; current chest pain considered due to myocardial ischemia; use of nitrate therapy; ECG with pathological Q waves
3 *History of congestive heart failure*: pulmonary edema, bilateral rales or S3 gallop; paroxysmal nocturnal dyspnea; CXR showing pulmonary vascular redistribution
4 *History of cerebrovascular disease*: prior TIA or stroke
5 *Pre-operative treatment with insulin*
6 *Pre-operative creatinine* > 2 mg/dL–176.8 μmol/L

score of Goldman et al. (1977) and Lee et al. (1999): Revised Cardiac Risk Index-RCRI (Table 11.2), which was prepared and tested in different populations (Ford et al. 2010). This score has a good ability to predict cardiovascular complications during non-cardiac surgery but its ability to predict cardiovascular mortality is not as accurate (Ford et al. 2010). The predictive value of this score in another interesting recent work seems to be frankly improved is associated with the measurement of NT-proBNP and CRP (Choi et al. 2010). This score seen from the geriatric perspective has some fundamental limitations: at first, often elderly heart patients in the post intervention die of non-cardiovascular death; second, in geriatric patients use the creatinine level to assess renal function is fallacious (Fig. 11.1).

About cardio surgical risk scores, currently between risk score used in clinical practice and tested in the literature we find the European System of Cardiac Operative Risk Evaluation (EuroSCORE) I (Roques et al. 1999) and II (Nashef et al. 2012) and the score of the Society of Thoracic Surgeons (STS) (Ferguson TB Jr et al. 2000). These risk scores provide relatively good discriminative capacity, adequate capacity to distinguish the layer of low-risk patients from the high risk. However, there are still significant differences between the expected risk and that observed, in particular for the EuroSCORE, which, compared with the STS, also tends to overestimate of two or three times the risk of mortality for cardiac surgery in adults compared to the actual mortality seen in clinical practice, especially in older and complex patients (Wendt et al. 2009). This appears even truer in patients undergoing cardiac valve surgery, in relation to the fact that these risk models have been developed and validated in cardiosurgical populations for the most part composed of individual patients undergoing CABG (Collart et al. 2005; Barili et al. 2010).

The EuroSCORE was developed in 1999 using the information regarding risk factors and mortality of 19,030 patients undergoing elective coronary artery bypass in 1995 in 128 European cardiac surgery centres. The score predicts the risk of death at 30 days in the form of logistic EuroSCORE (i.e. as a percentage risk) or as an additive EuroSCORE (<3 low risk, 3–6 medium risk or >6 high risk). However, among the 19,030 patients originally considered, only 3200 (17%) have been subjected, for example, also in aortic valve replacement. The score was therefore

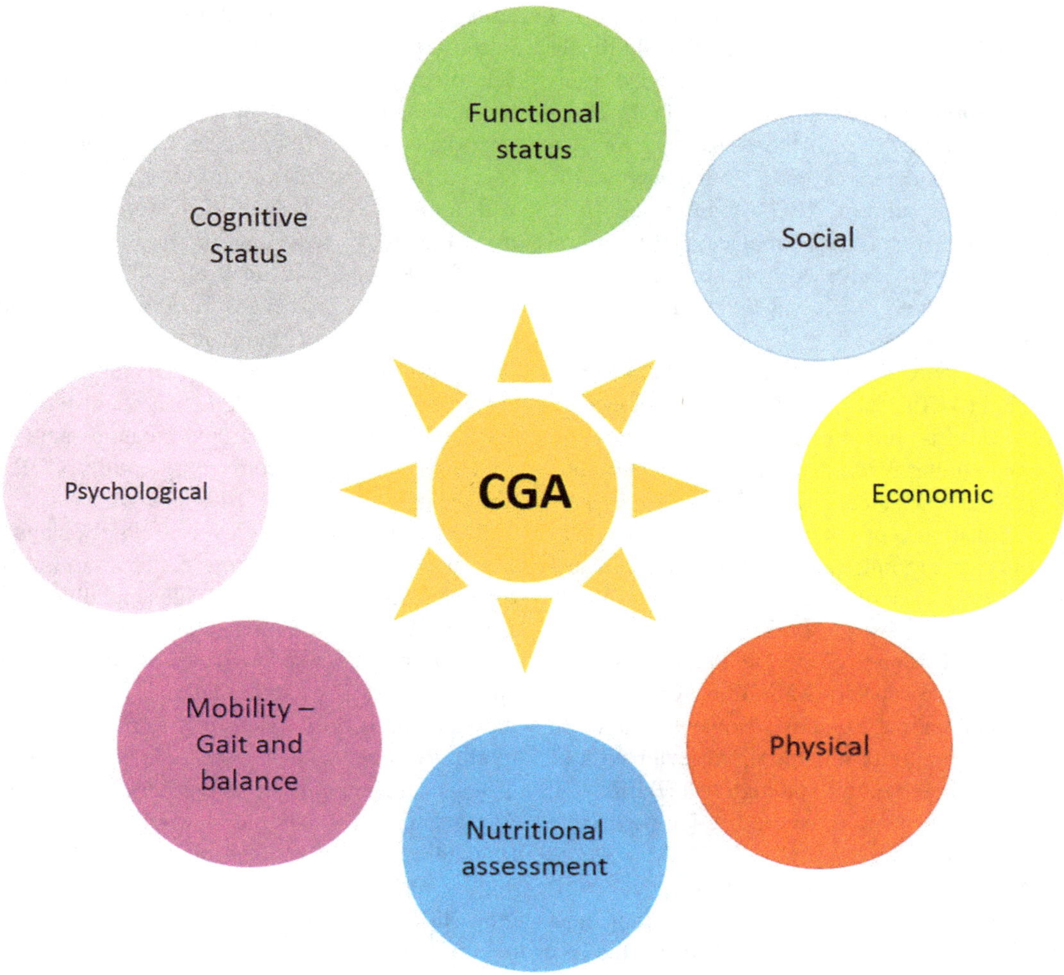

Fig. 11.1 Comprehensive geriatric assessment

developed assuming the intervention of single CABG as the basic risk model, while the action of the valve is considered as "other than CABG procedures". Therefore, the mitral and aortic valve replacement or mitral plastic, either alone or in combination with CABG, all fall in the same risk profile (Roques et al. 1999). In order to overcome the limitations of logistical and additive EuroSCORE, the EuroSCORE II was developed, more complex than the previous version, in spite of the risk factors considered are substantially the same (Nashef et al. 2012), and that has improved the evaluation of risk of several interventions by the single CABG. Despite such improvements, although the EuroSCORE II is still not one convincing score, especially in the evaluation of more complex patients and therefore at greater risk (Barili et al. 2013).

The STS score is a risk model developed by the Society of Thoracic Surgeons on the basis of demographic and clinical data in the adult population and is used for predicting the risk of operative mortality and morbidity after cardiac surgery. Compared all EuroSCORE, the STS is based on a large collection of data from more than 100,000 patients, taking into consideration morbidity outcomes (risk of revision surgery, stroke, acute renal failure, prolonged ventilation and hospitalization, surgical wound infection), it is periodically updated and a significantly higher number of valvular patients were included in his initial formulation (Ferguson et al. 2000). However, this model is realistic exclusively for procedures considered as case studies within the same model (single CABG; single aortic valve replacement, mitral valve replacement or mitral plastic; CABG+ valve one of the above procedures) effectively excluding interventions more complex surgical.

A new score, the Age, Creatinine and Ejection Fraction (ACEF) has recently been developed on the basis of a limited number of risk factors and showed similar results in terms of accuracy than EuroSCORE (Ranucci et al. 2009), but a most discrimination, primarily to the benefit of patients undergoing single aortic valve replacement (Ranucci et al. 2011).

Among these three score (STS, EuroSCORE II and ACEF) the STS has a greater discriminative capacity while EuroSCORE has a better calibration capacity. However, none of these three score is reliable in the evaluation of patients at intermediate and high risk (Barili et al. 2013), and even less to predict the long-term risk (Collart et al. 2005).

Particularly when applied in very old individual patient, these risk scores show their most important limits. This is mainly because the risk is not specific for the age group and is not well stratified, as already said, for the different interventions and for the various pathologies. Finally, many variables are not considered by any score (i.e. liver function, irradiation, fragility, etc.). These considerations reduce the reliability of these score, which need integration of new variables in the elderly population.

11.3 The Role of Comorbidity, Functional Status and *Frailty* in Surgery Risk Stratification

Comorbidity is defined as the simultaneous presence of two or more diseases in the same patient, an event that grows with increasing age and changes phenotype, whereas in the elderly comorbidities are usually chronical contrary that in the young (Abete et al. 2004). From the epidemiological point of view, the problem of chronic comorbidities in the elderly is very important but its clinical effects even more, because a significant comorbidity is associated with a higher risk of death (Librero et al. 1999), to a high risk of rehospitalisation, disability and poor quality of life (Chin et al. 1999).

Comorbidity influences the diagnostic and therapeutic process because often the coexistence of several diseases makes difficult the interpretation of symptoms and signs that characterize a disease. It is a classic example breathlessness of an elderly suffering from heart failure, COPD and anemia.

The high comorbidity level of elderly plays a central role in excluded these patients in clinical trials (Cherubini et al. 2010). Substantially in the most of geriatric cardiology studies, comorbidity it is simply assessed as disease count; this approach shows great limitations, especially if the outcome is not limited only to mortality and morbidity, but considers the risk of becoming disabled. Marchionni et al. (1996) had clearly demonstrated that in elderly individuals with heart failure the risk of becoming disabled was high due to the presence of the disease index but grew differently if it was associated with COPD or cerebrovascular disease; in the first association the risk of disability progressed substantially in order arithmetically, in the second case exponentially. The work well demonstrated as the interrelationship in terms of risk between two chronic conditions were much more complex than the simple sum of the risks and it was largely due to pathophysiological mechanisms, above all functional, confirming the fallacy of the approach disease count-type.

Finally, the evaluation of co-morbidity of the elderly has to include the measure of severity of individual diseases associated. Among many studies, the ICED-Index of coexisting disease Greenfield (Greenfield et al. 1993) and the Geriatric Index of Comorbidity-GIC (Rozzini et al. 2002) are to mention. The first one index predicts the risk of disability in patients suffering from chronic disease and consists of two subscales: one composed of a list of fourteen chronic conditions with clinical severity increasing from 0 to 4 and with the possibility to classify also diseases not on the list; the second subscale includes twelve domains in which the functional disability is scalable from 0 to 2. The ICED was validated in eight populations including in patients with myocardial infarction or coronary artery bypass grafting (Imamura et al. 1997). The GIC consists in a list of fifteen diseases with severity grading from 0 to 4, with the possibility to build four classes of comorbidity basing on the presence of one or more diseases associated (Rozzini et al. 2002).

While these scores are certainly able to better characterize the value and the level of comorbidity with respect to a count of associated diseases, we have to emphasize that in many chronic elderly diseases there is a dichotomy between symptom severity and prognosis, risk of death and risk of disability. This geriatric paradox is well explained by severe osteoarthritis, in which is obvious that the risk of becoming disabled is high when the joint symptoms is poorly controlled by drugs but the risk of death appears to be rather negligible.

The association between the elderly patient and surgical risk cannot exclude the integrity of global functional status. The global functional status is the capable of the whole of physical and cognitive abilities of an elderly to maintain the ability to perform normal activities of daily living and to maintain sufficient social network. This concept was measurable medicine geriatrics by the BADL (Basic Activities of Daily Living) (Katz et al. 1963) and IADL (Instrumental Activities of Daily Living) (Lawton and Brody 1969) scales.

The predictive value of this scale in geriatric medicine has a solid literature. Fukuse et al. (2005) showed that in older patients underwent thoracic surgery, a reduction of autonomy, measured by the number of BADL lost, is able to predict major perioperative complications, independent of other risk factors.

The probability of exit disabled by surgery is complicated by the difficulty to capture in the pre-operative the level of physiological homeostatic reserves and the vulnerability to stressful events that sums up the concept of *frailty* (Fukuse et al. 2005). The conceptual definition of *frailty* appears much discussed in geriatric medicine (Partridge and Harari 2012). Campbell defines *frailty* as "a condition or syndrome which results from a multi-system reduction in reserve capacity to the extent that a number of physiological systems are close to, or past, the threshold of symptomatic clinical failure" (Campbell and Buchner 1997).

Given this definition, there are two models of *frailty* suitable for the stratification of surgical risk of the elderly. They are summarized in the model called "Frailty phenotype" arising from the Cardiovascular Health Study (Fried et al. 2001) and in the "Deficit accumulation model of frailty" created by the Canadian Study of Health and Aging (Rockwood et al. 2001). The first substantially recognizes a set of five domains: unintentional weight loss, muscle strength measured by hand grip, the feeling of self-reported exhaustion, walking speed, the amount of physical activity habitual self-reported (Fried et al. 2001). The Canadian model builds a *frailty* index from a list of over 70 both functional and clinical items, exploring the physical, cognitive and disability in daily life, scoring from 0 to 7 for increasing fragility (Rockwood et al. 2001). Both models have been tested in the stratification of surgical risk of elderly patients proving ability to predict long-term adverse outcomes (Partridge and Harari 2012), but certainly showing some limitations related to the complexity of their implementation in clinical routine.

In our opinion, the assessment of the surgical risk of elderly should be take into account two key points: tools used have to be simple, reproducible and acceptable because of the complexity of the surgical setting; two, scores have to be able to stratify perioperative risk as well as to identify any modifiable factors to improved outcome (Partridge and Harari 2012).

Therefore it is useful in a preoperative setting rely patient assessment on surrogate, but quite reliable, measures of *frailty* such as physical performance tests. The strength of the upper limbs measured with the dynamometer (Handgrip test) or the gait speed performed in a short corridor are tools that have proved their worth in the field of surgical stratification of elderly patients (Makary et al. 2010; Klidjian et al. 1980). The attention to the measures of physical performance in the field of geriatric cardiology and cardiac surgery has significantly increased in recent years. Di Bari et al. have shown (Chiarantini et al. 2010) that the Short Physical Performance Battery (Guralnik et al. 1994) is able to predict independently the prognosis of elderly patients with heart failure as much as the NYHA class. Until recently, the group of DUKE University of Afilalo et al. (2010) has demonstrated as in 131 elderly undergoing cardiac surgery the speed along a corridor 5 m higher than 6 s identified a subpopulation at higher independent risk of mortality and morbidity. The risk is 2–3 times higher for each level of the STS score (STS Adult Cardiac Surgery Database Risk Model Variables—Data Version 2005) used for surgical preoperative screening by cardiac surgeons.

11.4 The Role of Comprehensive Geriatric Assessment (CGA) in Preoperative Cardiac Surgery

The rapid increase in the number of elderly people and life expectancy is accompanied by an increased demand for cardiac surgery in these patients, so much so that one of the most important and current topics in cardiology and geriatrics is represented by the difficult choice whether to submit or not elderly cardiac surgery. In fact, for this type of intervention, the current risk prediction models have poor performance and inaccurate in elderly patients, generally tending to overestimate the operative risk (Dupuis 2008). Nevertheless, the perception that these patients have a lower functional reserves and the fact that present greater comorbidity, made cardiologists and cardiac surgeons often hesitate to propose to elderly cardiac surgery. Despite the increase of co-morbidity in the elderly population undergoing cardiac surgery (increased incidence of diabetes, dyslipidemia, hypertension, and left main disease), mortality reported in the literature relative to octogenarians has been greatly reduced, with the downsizing of incidence of post-operative complications such as stroke, acute dysfunction of the pump and use of aortic counter pulsation (Maganti et al. 2009). Cardiac surgical procedures can be performed safely and with therapeutic benefit even in carefully selected nonagenarians (Ullery et al. 2008; Assmann et al. 2013). A recent study (Buth et al. 2014) analysed the variations of the type of population and the type of intervention in clinical practice in the last decade. Regarding the types of interventions, there has been a reduction of isolated CABG procedures and to an increase of the interventions on valve (mostly due to the increase of the aortic valve replacements) and of intervention on thoracic aorta or of device plant ventricular Assist; interventions combined CABG/valve were stable. As regards the age of the population operated, there has been a reduction of patients with <70 years and an increase in those >80 years of age; there were no significant changes in patients with ages between 70 and 79 years. The average age has grown in 10 years from 64.1 years to 65.4. There has also been an increase in the percentage of frail patients, in all three decades old, but the most significant among the over-eighties. Just among older and frail patients recorded a significant increase in the total hospital stay and intensive care unit stay. Also among frail patients, compared to non-brittle, even mortality and institutionalization they were much more frequent. Several studies, however, have shown how to foreclose the subject senior cardiac surgery only in relation to their age is not justified, because the elderly receive comparable benefits compared to younger in terms of symptoms, function and quality of life (Likosky et al. 2008; Zingone et al. 2009). In order to maximize the benefit of surgery for the elderly, however, it is necessary to be able to improve the selection of subjects to be subjected to surgery.

In 1991, the lack in management of elderly patients led to the development of a specific geriatric tool: the Comprehensive Geriatric Assessment (CGA) . This consists in a "*multidimensional interdisciplinary diagnostic process focused on determining a frail elderly person's medical, psychological and functional capability in order to develop a coordinated and integrated plan for treatment and long term follow up*" (Rubenstein et al. 1991).

From 1991 a growing interest has been demonstrating in the applicability and effectiveness of this tool in predict and prevent complications in cardiac and non-cardiac surgery. This includes assessment of medical, psychiatric, functional and socio-economical domains followed by a tailored management plan including rehabilitation; the team includes as a minimum experienced medical, nursing and therapy staff. The evaluation consists of administering standardised assessment tools to gather information in a semi-structured way. For example, this might include Basic and Instrumental Activities of Daily Living for functional evaluation (Katz et al. 1963), Geriatric Depression Scale for psychological screening (Sheikh and Yesavage 1986) or the Mini Mental State Examination for cognition (Folstein et al. 1975).

Only few studies incorporated disabilities in activities of daily living as a predictor of outcomes after cardiac surgery (Maillet et al. 2009; Lee et al. 2010).

A good test for the identification of elderly who, for reduced physical performance, are considered frail and therefore a high prognostic risk tool is the Short Physical Performance Battery (SPPB). The SPPB consists of three timed physical performance tests (walking speed, rising from a chair and balance), each with a score from 0 to 4: a total score of 5 out of 12 identifies the frail elderly. The marks obtained at SPPB is a powerful predictor of mortality in the elderly population, even after adjusting for age, sex, levels of multimorbidity and cognitive status (Guralnik et al. 1994; 1995).

In contrast to scales as the SPPB, which are composed of multiple items, the gait-speed and the measurement of the upper limb strength through dynamometer are measurable indicators of fragility as single items (Abellan van Kan et al. 2009; Dumurgier et al. 2009; Ling et al. 2010). The walking speed has been shown to have excellent reproducibility, intra- and inter-investigator. Furthermore, it is not so important the distance walked, which can vary in the different tests from 3 to 10 m, as the time to cover every meter (Graham et al. 2008). However, the distance of 5 m is the one most used, as it takes into account the possible occurrence of cardiopulmonary symptoms for longer paths. For each increment of 0.1 m/s of gait-speed there has been a reduction of approximately 12% risk of death (Studenski et al. 2011). A patient with a walking speed lower than 0.8 m/s is at greater risk of loss of autonomy, declining health status and increased risk of institutionalization and death (Studenski et al. 2003; Guralnik et al. 2000).

Up until only a few years ago, there were no studies specifically focusing on the use of gait speed as a predictor of post-operative mortality and morbidity in elderly cardiac surgery patients. A forerunner study in this field was conducted by Afilalo et al. (2010), in 131 patients undergoing cardiac surgery of 70 years of age or older (mean age of 75.8 ± 4.4 years). 46% of patients were defined as slow walkers (time to walk 5 m of $\geq$ 6 s] before cardiac surgery. The primary end point verified in 23% of patients (composite of in-hospital postoperative mortality or major morbidity). Slow gait speed has been demonstrated independently predict the composite endpoint after adjusting for the STS risk score (odds ratio: 3.05; 95% CI: 1.23–7.54). A subsequent study of Afilalo confirmed these results: slow walking and presence of high-level disability (at least 3 impairments in Nagi's scale) were associated with a significant increase in adjusted risk. Among the risk scores evaluated, the Parsonnet score and STS-PROMM demonstrated the best discriminative ability for mortality or major morbidity in elderly patients (Afilalo et al. 2012).

Another interesting study (Lee et al. 2010) defined *frailty* as any impairment in activities of daily living ambulation, or a documented history of dementia. Of 3826 patients, 157 (4.1%) were frail. Frail patients were older, were more likely to be female, and had risk factors for adverse surgical outcomes. By logistic regression, *frailty* was an independent predictor of in-hospital mortality (odds ratio 1.8; 95% CI: 1.1–3.0), as well as institutional discharge (odds ratio 6.3; 95% CI: 4.2–9.4) and of reduced midterm survival (hazard ratio 1.5; 95% CI: 1.1–2.2)

Sündermann et al. (2011) tested a more complex evaluation tool, called Comprehensive Assessment of Frailty (CAF). It included: unintentional weight loss; weakness (handgrip at dynamometer); self-reported exhaustion (through a specific Questionnaire); slowness of gait speed (time to walk 4 m); low activity (IADL); the evaluation of standing balance; a test to assess body control; laboratory tests (serum albumin, creatinine and Brain Natriuretic Peptide); measure of Forced Expiratory Volume in 1 s (FEV1) was measured. This protocol was applied to 400 patients ≥ 74 years. Median *frailty* score was 11; median of logistic EuroSCORE was 8.5% and of STS score was 3.3%. There was a significant correlation between *frailty* score and observed 30-day mortality ($P < 0.05$). The evident limit of this study was the complexity of the evaluation, which makes impossible apply it to real life. Fortunately, the same study group simplified the assessment and created the "Frailty predicts death One yeaR after Elective Cardiac Surgery Test (FORECAST)" (Sündermann et al. 2011), limited to the more predictable variables. These resulted: Chair rise (patient gets up and down from a chair three times and time is measured); Weak (in the last two weeks); stair (patient climbs as many stairs as he is able to); Clinical Frailty Scale (as estimated from one cardiac surgeon and an experienced clinician); creatinine. At one-year follow up, mortality rate was 12.2%. Patients who died within one year had a median *frailty* score of 16 compared to 11 to the one-year survivors ($P = 0.001$).

Another interesting practical implication of multidimensional geriatric evaluation is the ability to identify patients at high risk of developing delirium during hospitalization. Rudolph et al. (2009) recently published a paper on the development and validation of a scoring system to predict delirium after cardiac surgery, as defined by the Confusion Assessment Method (Inouye et al. 1990). They enrolled 122 elderly cardiac surgery patients that underwent a delirium assessment pre- and postoperatively beginning on postoperative day 2. Delirium occurred in 52% of the patients and multivariate analysis identified four independent variables associated with delirium: previous stroke, MMSE scores, abnormal serum albumin, and the geriatric Depression Scale scores.

11.5 The Role of Comprehensive Geriatric Assessment (CGA) in Interventional Cardiology

Older patients requiring PCI are more likely to have complex, multivessel disease often associated with altered hemostasis, platelet hyper-reactivity and blood hyper-viscosity, all factors increasing the risk of early thrombosis, or of dual antiplatelet therapy-related bleeding complications (Madhavan et al. 2018). Moreover, non-cardiac, comorbid conditions commonly encountered in advanced age (e.g.: chronic kidney disease with higher risk of contrast-induced nephropathy; even minor cognitive impairment increasing the likelihood of delirium), substantially increase the risk of adverse periprocedural outcomes in older candidates to PCI (Madhavan et al. 2018).

Interestingly Singh et al. demonstrated in a large cohort of elderly patients underwent PCI, the addition of frailty and comorbidity measure to the traditional cardiovascular risk factors improves risk prediction of older patients after PCI. Among 628 discharged older patients the three-year mortality was 28% for frail patients, 6% for nonfrail ones; after adjustment, frailty (HR = 4.19, 95% CI; 1.85–9.51), physical component score of the SF-36 (HR = 1.59; 95% CI; 1.24–2.02), and comorbidity, (HR = 1.10; 95% CI; 1.05–1.16) were independently associated with mortality. In addition introducing these variables in the model about 40% patients were moved to the higher risk category according to Mayo Clinic Risk Score definition (Singh et al.

2011). Murali-Krishnan R et al. demonstrated in 745 patients underwent PCI that the presence of frailty, defined according to Rockwood accumulation deficits score (Murali-Krishnan et al. 2015) was associated with increased 30-day (HR 4.8, 95% CI 1.4–16.3, $p = 0.013$) and 1 year mortality (HR 5.9, 95% CI 2.5–13.8, $p < 0.001$). In addition frailty was a predictor of length of hospital stay independent of age, gender and comorbidities.

In the field of valvular disease, a recent advent of transcatheter aortic valve implantation (TAVI) and its impressive worldwide utilization reports a clear shift for treating patients with severe aortic stenosis previously deemed inoperable or refused from different surgical procedures (Leon et al. 2010) and now, through recent data of the PARTNER program, patients considered at high (Smith et al. 2011) or intermediate (Leon et al. 2016) STS surgery risk can be eligible to this interventional procedure with non inferiority result respect to cardiac surgery and recently also in patients defined as low risk ones (Mack et al. 2019).

In the perspective of future increase of elderly patients candidates to TAVI, important efforts must be made to improve the prognostic ability of the current risk scores to capture short long term mortality and disability, and helping to resolve a crucial issue providing solid clinical indications to help physician in the definition of this interventional approach as futile.

Wendt et al., compared different risk scoring algorithms on isolated conventional or transcatheter aortic valve implantation and certified how the predictive value of many currently available risk-scoring algorithms is insufficient to allow a precise and reliable risk assessment in patients undergoing surgical aortic valve replacement or TAVI, with the result of overestimation for logistic EuroSCORE-I and a clear underestimation of the risk for the Society of Thoracic Surgeons (STS) score logistic EuroSCORE-II and age-creatinine-ejection fraction (ACEF) score (Chakos et al. 2017). These authors highlighted how frailty and comorbidity are the most significant missing parameters not evaluated by traditional risk scores and their incorporation in newly scores must to be considered as a mandatory challenge in the next future.

In support of this clinical view, recent data confirm the crucial role of Comprehensive Geriatric Assessment-CGA as a predictor of prognosis after transcatheter aortic valve Implantation (Stortecky et al. 2012). In fact Stortecky et al. in a prospective cohort of 100 consecutive patients aged equal or more 70 years undergoing TAVI, risk prediction can be substantially improved the prognostic power of recommended risk scores by adding MGA based informations such as cognitive level, malnutrition, frailty index, and impairment in activities of daily living.

Schoenenberger et al. (2013) prospectively demonstrated that an index of frailty strongly predicted post-TAVI functional decline when adjusted for both the STS and EuroSCOREs; in addition data showed, over a 6-month period, that functional status worsened only in a minority of patients surviving TAVI. Indeed in this study the frailty index was a mixed association of frailty and disability parameters because it was calculated as summary score (from 0 to 7) from the following baseline components: MMSE, TUG, MNA, BADL limited activity, IADL limited activity, and a pre-clinical mobility disability (defined as decreased frequency of walking 200 m and/or of climbing stairs during the preceding 6 months).

Similarly Green et al. recently reported on a PARTNER substudy evaluating the prognostic value of frailty (assessed using a composite of albumin levels, dominant handgrip strength, gait speed, and Katz index) in older TAVI recipients. They demonstrated in 244 patients of the study population that all-cause mortality rate was 32.7% in the frail group and 15.9% in the non-frail group (log-rank $p < 0.004$). At 1 year, poor outcome included 30-day cardiac death, repeat hospitalization because of AS or complications of the valve procedure, stroke, major bleeding, major vascular complications, permanent pacemaker, and renal failure requiring dialysis occurred in 50.0% of the frail group and 31.5% of the nonfrail group (p = 0.02) Relation between six-minute walk test performance and outcomes after transcatheter aortic valve implantation (from the PARTNER trial) (Green et al. 2013).

Although at present, substantial differences can be detected among instruments utilized for measuring frailty in patients candidate to TAVI, The AHA/ACC guidelines on managing patients with valvular heart disease support frailty measuring when assessing peri-procedural risk because this additive evaluation will likely optimize the selection of TAVI candidates could have the maximal benefit from the procedure.

References

Abellan van Kan G, Rolland Y, Andrieu S, Bauer J, Beauchet O, Bonnefoy M et al (2009) Gait speed at usual pace as a predictor of adverse ut comes in community-dwelling older people: an International Academy on Nutrition and Aging (IANA) Task Force. J Nutr Health Aging 13:881–889

Abete P, Testa G, Della Morta D, Mazzella F, Galizia G, D'Ambrosio D et al (2004) La comorbilità nell'anziano: epidemiologia e caratteristiche cliniche. G Gerontol 52:267–272

Afilalo J, Eisenberg MJ, Morin JF, Bergman H, Monette J, Noiseux N et al (2010) Gait speed as an incremental predictor of mortality and major morbidity in elderly patients undergoing cardiac surgery. J Am Coll Cardiol 56:1668–1676

Afilalo J, Mottillo S, Eisenberg MJ, Alexander KP, Noiseux N, Perrault LP et al (2012) Addition of frailty and disability to cardiac surgery risk scores identifies elderly patients at high risk of mortality or major morbidity. Circ Cardiovasc Qual Outcomes 5:222–228

American Society of Anesthesiologists (1963) New classification of physical status. Anesthesiology 24:111

American Society of Anesthesiologists. ASA Physical Status Classification System (2014) Web. 26 Luglio 2019. https://www.asahq.org/standards-and-guidelines/asa-physical-status-classification-system

Assmann A, Minol JP, Mehdiani A, Akhyari P, Boeken U et al (2013) Cardiac surgery in nonagenarians: not only feasible, but also reasonable? Interact CardioVasc Thorac Surg 17:340–343

Association of Anaesthetists of Great Britain and Ireland (2014) Perioperative care of the elderly 2014. Anaesthesia 69:81–98

Barili F, Di Gregorio O, Capo A, Ardemagni E, Rosato F, Argenziano M et al (2010) Aortic valve replacement: reliability of EuroSCORE in predicting early outcomes. Int J Cardiol 144:343–345

Barili F, Pacini D, Capo A, Rasovic O, Grossi C, Alamanni F et al (2013) Does EuroSCORE II perform better than its original versions? a multicentre validation study. Eur Heart J 34:22–29

Barnett S, Moonesinghe SR (2011) Clinical risk scores to guide perioperative management. Postgrad Med J 87:535–541

Bennett-Guerrero E, Hyam JA, Shaefi S, Prytherch DR, Sutton GL, Weaver PC et al (2003) Comparison of P-POSSUM risk adjusted mortality rates after surgery between patients in the USA and the UK. Br J Surg 90:1593–1598

Buth KJ, Gainer RA, Legare JF, Hirsch GM (2014) The changing face of cardiac surgery: practice patterns and outcomes 2001–2010. Can J Cardiol 30:224–230

Campbell AJ, Buchner DM (1997) Unstable disability and the fluctuations of frailty. Age Ageing 26:315–318

Chakos A, Wilson-Smith A, Arora S, Nguyen TC, Dhoble A, Tarantini G et al (2017) Long term outcomes of transcatheter aortic valve implantation (TAVI): a systematic review of 5-year survival and beyond. Ann Cardiothorac Surg 6:432–443

Cherubini A, Del Signore S, Ouslander J, Semla T, Michel JP (2010) Fighting against age discrimination in clinical trials. J Am Geriatr Soc 58:1791–1796

Chiarantini D, Volpato S, Fotini S, Bartalucci F, Del Bianco L, Mangani I et al (2010) Lower extremity performance measures predict long-term prognosis in older patients hospitalized for heart failure. J Card Fail 16:390–395

Chin MH, Jin L, Karrison TG Mulliken R, Hayley DC, Walter J et al (1999) Older patients health-related quality of life around an episode of emergency illness. Ann Emerg Med 54:595–601

Choi J-H, Cho DK, Song Y-B, Hahn JY, Choi S, Gwon HC et al (2010) Preoperative NT-proBNP and CRP predict perioperative major cardiovascular events in non-cardiac surgery. Heart 96:56–62

Chow WB, Rosenthal RA, Merkow RP, Ko CY, Esnaola NF (2012) Optimal preoperative assessment of the geriatric surgical patient: a best practices guideline from the American College of Surgeons National Surgical Quality Improvement Program and the American Geriatrics Society. J Am Coll Surg 215:453–466

Collart F, Feier H, Kerbaul F, Mouly-Bandini A, Riberi A, Mesana TG et al (2005) Valvular surgery in octogenarians: operative risks factors, evaluation of Euroscore and long term results. Eur J Cardiothorac Surg 27:276–280

Copeland GP, Jones D, Waters M (1991) POSSUM: a scoring system for surgical audit. Br J Surg 78:355–360

Dumurgier J, Elbaz A, Ducimetière P, Tavernier B, Alpérovitch A, Tzourio C (2009) Slow walking speed and cardiovascular death in well functioning older adults: prospective cohort study. BMJ 339:4460

Dupuis JY (2008) Predicting outcomes in cardiac surgery: risk stratification matters? Curr Opin Cardiol 23:560–567

Ellis G, Spiers M, Coutts S, Fairburn P, McCracken L (2012) Preoperative assessment in the elderly: evaluation of a new clinical service. Scott Med J 57:212–216

Etzioni DA, Liu JH, Maggard MA, Ko CY (2003) The aging population and its impact on the surgery workforce. Ann Surg 238:170–177

Ferguson TB Jr, Dziuban SW Jr, Edwards FH, Eiken MC, Shroyer AL, Pairolero PC et al (2000) The STS national database: current changes and challenges for the new millennium. Committee to establish a national database in cardiothoracic surgery, The Society of Thoracic Surgeons. Ann Thorac Surg 69:680–91

Folstein MF, Folstein SE, McHugh PR (1975) "Mini-mental state". A practical method for grading the cognitive state of patients for the clinician. J Psychiatr Res 12:189–98

Ford MK, Beattie SW, Wijeysundera DN (2010) Systematic review: prediction of perioperative cardiac complications and mortality by the revised cardiac risk index. Ann Intern Med 152:26–35

Fried LP, Tangen CM, Walston J, Newman AB, Hirsch C, Gottdiener J et al (2001) Frailty in older adults: evidence for a phenotype. J Gerontol A Biol Sci Med Sci 56:146–156

Fukuse T, Satoda N, Hijiya K, Fujinaga T (2005) Importance of comprehensive geriatric assessment in prediction of complications following thoracic surgery in elderly patients. Chest 127:886–891

Goldman L, Caldera DL, Nussbaum SR, Southwick FS, Krogstad D, Murray B et al (1977) Multifactorial index of cardiac risk in noncardiac surgical procedures. N Engl J Med 297:845–850

Goldstein LJ, Halpern JA, Rezayat C, Gallagher KA, Sambol EB, Bush HL Jr et al (2010) Endovascular aneurysm repair in nonagenarians is safe and effective. J Vasc Surg 52:1140–1146

Graham JE, Ostir GV, Kuo Y-F, Fisher SR, Ottenbacher KJ (2008) Relationship between test methodology and mean velocity in timed walk tests: a review. Arch Phys Med Rehabil 89:865–872

Green P, Cohen DJ, Généreux P, McAndrew T, Arnold SV, Alu M et al (2013) Relation between six-minute walk test performance and outcomes after transcatheter aortic valve implantation (from the PARTNER trial). Am J Cardiol 112:700–706

Greenfield S, Apolone G, McNeil BJ, Cleary PD (1993) The importance of co-existent disease in the occurrence of postoperative complications and one-year recovery in patients undergoing total hip replacement. Comorbidity and outcomes after hip replacement. Med Care 31:141–154

Guralnik JM, Simonsick EM, Ferrucci L, Glynn RJ, Berkman LF, Blazer DG et al (1994) A short physical performance battery assessing lower extremity function: association with self-reported disability and prediction of mortality and nursing home admission. J Gerontol 49:85–94

Guralnik JM, Ferrucci L, Simonsick EM, Salive ME, Wallace RB (1995) Lower-extremity function in persons over the age of 70 years as a predictor of subsequent disability. N Engl J Med 332:556–562

Guralnik JM, Ferrucci L, Pieper CF, Leveille SG, Markides KS, Ostir GV et al (2000) Lower extremity function and subsequent disability: consistency across studies, predictive models, and value of gait speed alone compared with the short physical performance battery. J Gerontol A Biol Sci Med Sci 55:221–231

Harari D, Hopper A, Dhesi J, Babic-Illman G, Lockwood L, Martin F (2007) Proactive care of older people undergoing surgery ('POPS'): designing, embedding, evaluating and funding a comprehensive geriatric assessment service for older elective surgical patients. Age Ageing 36:190–196

Imamura K, McKinnon M, Middleton R, Black N (1997) Reliability of a comorbidity measure: the Index of Co-Existent Disease (ICED). J Clin Epidemiol 50:1011–1016

Inouye SK, Van Dyck CH, Alessi CA, Balkin S, Siegal AP, Horwitz RI (1990) Clarifying confusion: the confusion assessment method. A new method for detection of delirium. Ann Intern Med 113:941–948

Katz S, Ford AB, Moskowitz RW, Jackson BA, Jaffe MW (1963) Studies of illness in the aged, the index of ADL: a standardized measure of biological and psychosocial function. JAMA 185:914–919

Klidjian AM, Foster KJ, Kammerling RM, Cooper A, Karran SJ (1980) Relation of anthropometric and dynamometric variables to serious postoperative complications. Br Med J 281:899–901

Klopfenstein CE, Herrmann FR, Michel JP, Clergue F, Forster A (1998) The influence of an aging surgical population on the anesthesia workload: a ten-year survey. Anesth Analg 86:1165–1170

Kurian AA, Suryadevara S, Vaughn D, Zebley DM, Hofmann M, Kim S et al (2010) Laparoscopic colectomy in octogenarians and nonagenarians: a preferable option to open surgery? J Surg Educ 67:161–166

Lawton MP, Brody EM (1969) Self-maintaining and instrumental activities of daily living. Gerontologist. 9:179–186

Lee TH, Marcantonio ER, Mangione CM, Thomas EJ, Polanczyk CA, Cook EF et al (1999) Derivation and prospective validation of a simple index for prediction of cardiac risk of major noncardiac surgery. Circulation 100:1043–1049

Lee DH, Buth KJ, Martin BJ, Yip AM, Hirsch GM (2010) Frail patients are at increased risk for mortality and prolonged institutional care after cardiac surgery. Circulation 121:973–978

Leon MB, Smith CR, Mack MJ, Miller DG, Moses JW, Svensson LG et al (2010) Transcatheter aortic-valve implantation for aortic stenosis in patients who cannot undergo surgery. N Engl J Med 363:1597–1607

Leon MB, Smith CR, Mack MJ, Makkar RR, Svensson LG, Kodali SK et al (2016) Transcatheter or surgical aortic-valve replacement in intermediate-risk patients. N Engl J Med 374:1609–1620

Librero J, Peiró S, Ordiñana R (1999) Chronic comorbidity and outcomes of hospital care: length of stay, mortality, and readmission at 30 and 365 days. J Clin Epidemiol 52:171–179

Likosky DS, Dacey LJ, Baribeau YR, Leavitt BJ, Clough R, Cochran RP et al (2008) Group NNECDS. Long-term survival of the very elderly undergoing coronary artery bypass grafting. Ann Thorac Surg 85:1233–1237

Ling CHY, Taekema D, de Craen AJM, Gussekloo J, Westendorp RG, Maier AB (2010) Handgrip strength and mortality in the oldest old population: the Leiden 85-plus study. CMAJ 182:429–435

Mack MJ, Leon MB, Thourani VH, Makkar R, Kodali SK, Russo M et al (2019) Transcatheter aortic-valve replacement with a balloon-expandable valve in low-risk patients. N Engl J Med 380:1695–1705

Madhavan MV, Gersh BJ, Alexander KP, Granger CB, Stone GW (2018) Coronary Artery Disease in Patients $\geq$ 80 Years of Age. J Am Coll Cardiol 71:2015–2040

Maganti M, Rao V, Brister S, Ivanov J (2009) Decreasing mortality for coronary artery bypass surgery in octogenarians. Can J Cardiol 25:e32–e35

Maillet JM, Somme D, Hennel E, Lessana A, Saint-Jean O, Brodaty D (2009) Frailty after Aortic Valve Replacement (AVR) in octogenarians. Arch Gerontol Geriatr 48:391–396

Makary MA, Segev DL, Pronovost PJ, Syin D, Bandeen-Roche K, Patel P et al (2010) Frailty as a predictor of surgical outcomes in older patients. J Am Coll Surg 210:901–908

Marchionni N, Di Bari M, Fumagalli S, Ferrucci L, Baldereschi G, Timpanelli M et al (1996) Variable effect of comorbidity on the association of chronic cardiac failure with disability in community-dwelling older persons. Arch Gerontol Geriatr 23:283–292

Murali-Krishnan R, Iqbal J, Rowe R, Hatem E, Parviz Y, Richardson J et al (2015) Impact of frailty on outcomes after percutaneous coronary intervention: a prospective cohort study. Open Heart 2:1–6

Myles PS (2014) Meaningful outcome measures in cardiac surgery. J Extra Corpor Technol 46:23–27

Nakamura E, Miyao K (2007) A method for identifying biomarkers of aging and constructing an index of biological age in humans. J Gerontol A Biol Sci Med Sci 62:1096–1105

Nashef SA, Roques F, Sharples LD, Nilsson J, Smith C, Goldstone AR et al (2012) EuroSCORE II. Eur J Cardiothorac Surg 41:734–744

National Confidential Enquiry into Patient Outcome and Death (2010) An age old problem. A review of the care received by elderly patients undergoing surgery. NCEPOD, London

Naughton C, Feneck RO (2007) The impact of age on 6-month survival in patients with cardiovascular risk factors undergoing elective non-cardiac surgery. Int J Clin Pract 61:768–776

Partridge JSL, Harari D (2012) Frailty in the older surgical patient: a review. Age Ageing 41:142–147

Partridge J, Harari D, Martin F, Dhesi J (2014) The impact of preoperative comprehensive geriatric assessment on postoperative outcomes in older patients undergoing scheduled surgery: a systematic review. Anaesthesia 69:8–16

Polanczyk CA, Marcantonio E, Goldman L, Rohde LE, Orav J, Mangione CM et al (2001) Impact of age on perioperative complications and length of stay in patients undergoing noncardiac surgery. Ann Int Med 134:637–643

Prytherch DR, Whiteley MS, Higgins B, Weaver PC, Prout WG, Powell SJ (1998) POSSUM and Portsmouth POSSUM for predicting mortality. Physiological and operative severity score for the enumeration of mortality and morbidity. Br J Surg 85:1217–20

Ranucci M, Castelvecchio S, Menicanti L, Frigiola A, Pelissero G (2009) Risk of assessing mortality risk in elective cardiac operations: age, creatinine, ejection fraction, and the law of parsimony. Circulation 119:3053–3061

Ranucci M, Castelvecchio S, Conte M, Megliola G, Speziale G, Fiore F et al (2011) The easier, the better: age, creatinine, ejection fraction score for operative mortality risk stratification in a series of 29,659 patients undergoing elective cardiac surgery. J Thorac Cardiovasc Surg 142:581–586

Rockwood K, Wolfson C, McDowell I (2001) The Canadian study of health and aging: organizational lessons from a national, multicenter, epidemiologic study. Int Psychogeriatr 13:233–237

Roques F, Nashef SA, Michel P, Gauducheau E, De Vincentiis C, Baudet E et al (1999) Risk factors and outcome in European cardiac surgery: analysis of the EuroSCORE multinational database of 19030 patients. Eur J Cardiothorac Surg 15:816–822

Rozzini R, Frisoni GB, Ferrucci L Barbisoni P, Sabatini T, Ranieri P et al (2002) Geriatric index of comorbidity: validation and comparison with other measures of comorbidity. Age Ageing 31:277–285

Rubenstein LZ, Stuck AE, Siu AL, Wieland D (1991) Impacts of geriatric evaluation and management programs on defined outcomes: overview of the evidence. J Am Geriatr Soc 39:8S–16S

Rudolph JL, Jones RN, Levkoff SE, Rockett C, Inouye SK, Sellke FW et al (2009) Derivation and validation of a preoperative prediction rule for delirium after cardiac surgery. Circulation 119:229–236

Saklad M (1941) Grading of patients for surgical procedures. Anesthesiology 2:281–284

Schoenenberger AW, Stortecky S, Neumann S, Moser A, Jüni P, Carrel T et al (2013) Predictors of functional decline in elderly patients undergoing transcatheter aortic valve implantation (TAVI). Eur Heart J 34:684–692

Shahian DM, Edwards FH, Ferraris VA, Haan CK, Rich JB, Normand SL et al (2007) Quality measurement in adult cardiac surgery: part 1—conceptual framework and measure selection. Ann Thorac Surg 83:S3–S12

Sheikh JI, Yesavage JA (1986) Geriatric Depression Scale (GDS): recent evidence and development of a shorter version. Clin Gerontol 5:165–173

Singh M, Rihal CS, Lennon RJ, Spertus JA, Nair KS, Roger VL (2011) Influence of frailty and health status on outcomes in patients with coronary disease undergoing percutaneous revascularization. Circ Cardiovasc Qual Outcomes 4:496–502

Smith CR, Leon MB, Mack MJ, Miller DG, Moses JW, Svensson LG et al (2011) Transcatheter versus surgical aortic-valve replacement in high-risk patients. N Engl J Med 364:2187–2198

Stortecky S, Schoenenberger AW, Moser A, Kalesan B, Jüni P, Carrel T et al (2012) Evaluation of multidimensional geriatric assessment as a predictor of mortality and cardiovascular events after transcatheter aortic valve implantation. JACC Cardiovasc Interv 5:489–496

STS Adult Cardiac Surgery Database Risk Model Variables—Data Version 2.73 (2005–2012) The Society of Thoracic Surgeons

Studenski S, Perera S, Wallace D, Chandler JM, Duncan PW, Rooney E et al (2003) Physical performance measures in the clinical setting. J Am Geriatr Soc 51:314–322

Studenski S, Perera S, Patel K, Rosano C, Faulkner K, Inzitari M et al (2011) Gait speed and survival in older adults. JAMA 305:50–58

Sündermann S, Dademasch A, Praetorius J, Kempfert J, Dewey T, Falk V et al (2011a) Comprehensive assessment of frailty for elderly high-risk patients undergoing cardiac surgery. Eur J Cardiothorac Surg 39:33–37

Sündermann S, Dademasch A, Rastan A et al (2011b) One-year follow-up of patients undergoing elective cardiac surgery assessed with the comprehensive assessment of frailty test and its simplified form. Interact CardioVasc Thorac Surg 13:119–123

The Society of Thoracic Surgeons (2006) STS national database. Web. 26 Luglio 2019. https://www.sts.org/registries-research-center/sts-national-database

Ullery BW, Peterson JC, Milla F (2008) Cardiac surgery in select nonagenarians: should we or shouldn't we? Ann Thorac Surg 85:854–860

Wendt D, Osswald BR, Kayser K, Thielmann M, Tossios P, Massoudy P et al (2009) Society of Thoracic Surgeons Score is superior to the EuroSCORE determining mortality in high risk patients undergoing isolated aortic valve replacement. Ann Thorac Surg 88:468–474

Wolters U, Wolf T, Stutzer H, Schröder T, Pichlmaier H et al (1997) Risk factors, complications, and outcome in surgery: a multivariate analysis. Eur J Surg 163:563–568

Zingone B, Gatti G, Rauber E, Tiziani P, Dreas L, Pappalardo A et al (2009) Early and late outcomes of cardiac surgery in octogenarians. Ann Thorac Surg 87:71–78

Physical Exercise for Frailty and Cardiovascular Diseases

12

Natalia Aquaroni Ricci and Ana Izabel Lopes Cunha

Abstract

Cardiovascular diseases (CVD) and frailty syndrome are major problems for successful aging. These conditions share many biological aspects, symptoms and adverse effects. Aerobic capacity and muscle strength, that are important characteristics for independence in daily activity, are markedly reduced in older adults with CVD and frailty. There are evidence and recommendations of physical activity and exercises to prevent, treat and manage these conditions. However, the exact dose-response (type, intensity and duration) of exercises is still uncertain for these population. A good physical exercise program should consider the aging physiologic alterations, the vulnerability of the frail syndrome, and the functional-structural changes of CVD. Therefore, a multicomponent program with aerobic and strength training is desirable to improve these conditions. For long term results it is important to older adults with these conditions to change lifestyle and be more active during daily living to reduce sedentary behavior. Being frail with CVD it is not a contraindication for older adults to be engaged in physical activities.

Keywords

Frailty · Cardiovascular rehabilitation · Physical exercise

12.1 Introduction

Since the 21th century, the average lifespan is increasing worldwide. However, despite increased population longevity, there has been a rising burden of people living with chronic diseases and functional impairment (Prince et al. 2015; Viña et al. 2016). Much of this burden is attributable to an old recognized problem that is cardiovascular disease (Prince et al. 2015; Viña et al. 2016) and a relatively "new" phenomenon the frailty syndrome (García-Peña et al. 2016; Viña et al. 2016). It is common that older adults, especially those that are very old, share both conditions, cardiovascular disease and frailty syndrome (Nadruz et al. 2017; Vigorito et al. 2017).

Prevention and management of cardiovascular disease and frailty is essential. One intervention of considerable interest is physical activity and exercises. In this chapter we will present the importance of physical activity for healthy aging, for frailty and for cardiovascular diseases prevention and management. Also, the need for a special physical exercises approach when these conditions are presented simultaneous on older adults.

N. A. Ricci (✉) · A. I. L. Cunha
Universidade Cidade de São Paulo-UNICID, São Paulo, Brazil
e-mail: natalia_ricci@hotmail.com

N. Veronese (ed.), *Frailty and Cardiovascular Diseases*, Advances in Experimental Medicine and Biology 1216, https://doi.org/10.1007/978-3-030-33330-0_12

12.2 Physical Exercise for Healthy Aging

Typically, as people age, there is a decline in both physical activity and physical exercise levels, and therefore, an increase in physical inactivity and sedentary behavior. Physical activity is defined as any body movement produced by skeletal muscles contraction (Caspersen et al. 1985; ACSM 2009) that results in augmented of energy expenditure ≥ 1.5 METs (SBRN 2012), e.g. gardening, walking to grocery. While physical inactivity is being bellow recommendations of physical activity level, that is for older adults not achieving 150 min of moderate-to-vigorous-intensity physical activity per week (WHO 2010; SBRN 2012; González et al. 2017; Tremblay et al. 2017) . Physical exercise is a subset of physical activity that is planned, structured and repeated with the objective of improving or maintaining physical fitness (Caspersen et al. 1985), e.g. strength training. Sedentary behavior is defined as any wakeful behavior characterized by an energy expenditure ≤ 1.5 METs in posture lying, sitting or reclining (SBRN 2012; Tremblay et al. 2017), e.g. watching television, using the computer.

Inactivity and sedentary behavior are major contributors to morbidity and mortality among older adults (González et al. 2017; Perracini et al. 2017). Thus, physical activity plays an important role in healthy aging and to chronic disease management (Daskalopoulou et al. 2017). It is important to highlight that being active and the practice of regular physical exercises is not only a recommendation for robust older adults, but particularly imperative for those with chronic diseases, disabilities and frail (ACSM 2009; Perracini et al. 2017). Thus, physical training can be viewed as a preventive measure for the occurrence of chronic diseases or as a actual therapy to well-compensate and stable diseases (Pedersen and Saltin 2006). Table 12.1 displays the evidence regarding the practice of aerobic, strength, balance and stretching exercises for older adults (ACSM 2009; Elsawy and Higgins 2010).

There are several Recommendations- Guidelines for Physical Activity for older adults, Table 12.2 displays the most widespread ones (ACSM 2009; WHO 2010; Piercy et al. 2018).

Despite the evidence of the benefits of these recommendations for health, older adults find difficult to perform moderate and vigorous physical activity intensity (Matthews et al. 2008; Sparling et al. 2015). People aged 70–79 years old spend 9.6 h of their awake time in sedentary condition and less than 10–15% of older adults are meeting the minimum standard of >150 min/week of moderate intensity activity (Matthews et al. 2008). Fulfill these requirements can be even harder for those with multimorbidity, disabilities, frailty and chronic diseases. Nevertheless, the Guidelines state that for those older adults that cannot meet the amount or intensity of the exercises, they can still have benefits from engaging in physical activity less than those endorsed (Nelson et al. 2007; WHO 2010; Sparling et al. 2015; Piercy et al. 2018).

For sedentary older adults that want to start practicing physical exercise it is necessary to begin with light-intensity activity and the duration and number of days a week should increase slowly (Elsawy and Higgins 2010). For those with disability it is important to highlight that regular and oriented exercises is safe and can improve functional capacity and independence (Elsawy and Higgins 2010). And for those with an acute injury or illness a pause can be necessary, until the individual can get back to practice in a low level and increase slowly to the previous level (Elsawy and Higgins 2010).

Before initiating physical exercise practice, older adults with chronic health conditions, especially those with cardiac risk factors and physical limitations, should undergo pre-exercise evaluation (Elsawy and Higgins 2010). Absolute contraindications are just for moderate to high intensity activities and include recent myocardial infarction or electrocardiographic changes, complete heart block, unstable angina, uncontrolled hypertension, congestive heart failure (ACSM 2009; Elsawy and Higgins 2010). So, increasing

Table 12.1 Evidence of exercises in older adults

Type of Exercise	Level of evidence A	Level of evidence B
Aerobic training	Improve and maintain health: moderate intensity for at least 30 min on weekdays, or vigorous intensity for at least 20 min on 3 days-week (Elsawy and Higgins 2010) Increase VO_{2max}: intensity > 60% of VO_{2max} pre-training, 3 days-week for 16 weeks (ACSM 2009) Cardiovascular adaptations at rest: moderate-intensity aerobic exercises (ACSM 2009)	– Long-term vigorous intensity is associated with elevated cardiovascular reserve and skeletal muscle adaptations, which allow trained older adults to maintain a submaximal exercise load with less cardiovascular stress and muscle fatigue (ACSM 2009) – Prolonged aerobic exercise decreases age-related body fat accumulation, providing cardioprotective effect (ACSM 2009) – Promote metabolic adaptations, e.g. increasing glycemic control and lipid clearance (ACSM 2009) – Effective in combating age-related declines in bone density in postmenopausal women (ACSM 2009)
Resistance training	Increase strength and muscular power (ACSM 2009)	– At least 2 days-week for maintaining health and physical independence (Elsawy and Higgins 2010) – Prolonged strength training is associated with increased muscle mass and bone density (ACSM 2009) – High-intensity strength training is effective in treating clinical depression (ACSM 2009)
Balance training	Reduce the risk of falls and related injuries (Elsawy and Higgins 2010)	
Flexibility training		– At least 2 days—week for 10 min to maintain or increase the flexibility needed to practice physical activity and daily living activities (Elsawy and Higgins 2010)

Level A: consistent, good-quality patient-oriented evidence; level B: inconsistent or limited-quality patient-oriented evidence (Elsawy and Higgins 2010)
Level A: evidence from randomized clinical trials and/or observational studies with consistent results. Level B: evidence from randomized clinical trials and/or observational studies with some inconsistent results for the overall conclusion (ACSM 2009)

the daily activity, i.e., physical activity behavior, and exercises in low level has no contraindications for older people.

12.3 Physical Exercise for Frailty Syndrome

The frailty syndrome is defined as a state of vulnerability to adverse outcomes resulting from a decreased reserve and resistance to stressors (Fried et al. 2001). It is a dynamic state, i.e. can improve or worsen over time, in which one or more domains (physical, psychological and social) is affected (Gobbens et al. 2010a; Morley et al. 2013). Although all domains are important to the development of frailty, in its first conceptualization frailty phenotype was considered as an exclusively physical condition (Morley et al. 2013; de Labra et al. 2015). This physical phenotype consisting of five components: weight loss, exhaustion, weakness, low gait speed, and reduced physical activity (Fried et al. 2001; Morley et al. 2013). More recently, a consensus defined physical frailty as "a medical syndrome with multiple causes and contributors that is characterized by diminished strength, endurance, and reduced physiologic function that increases

Table 12.2 Recommendations—guidelines for physical activity for older adults

Recommendations	Population	Goal	Prescription
WHO—Global recommendations on Physical Activity for health (WHO 2010)	All individuals ≥ 65 years – Precautious and adjustments for those with chronic diseases and disabilities	– Improve cardiorespiratory, bone, muscular conditions and functional health; – Reduce mental illnesses (depression and cognitive disorders) and the risk of chronic disease	– Aerobic exercises: at least 150 min of moderate-intensity or 75 min of vigorous-intensity during the week, or an equivalent combination of moderate- and vigorous-intensity activity. For additional benefits, the above amount should be increased to 300 and 150 min respectively. The exercises should be performed in bouts of at least 10 min duration – Muscle-strengthening exercises: should involve major muscle groups on ≥ 2 days-week – To enhance balance and prevent falls physical activity should be performed on ≥ 3 days a week for those with poor mobility
The American College of Sports Medicine—Exercise and physical activity for older adults (ACSM 2009)	All individuals ≥ 65 years – Older adults with clinically significant chronic conditions or functional limitations	– Reduce the risk of chronic diseases, premature mortality, functional limitations and disabilities	– At least 150 min of physical activity per week – Aerobic exercises: minimum of 30 or up to 60 min of moderate-intensity on 5 days-week or a minimum of 20 or up to 30 min of vigorous-intensity 3 days-week, or an equivalent combination of moderate- and vigorous-intensity activity. Exercises should be in bouts of at least 10 min duration – Muscle-strengthening: at least 2 nonconsecutive days-week with a level of effort moderate to high and should involve major muscle groups – Flexibility exercises: 2 days-week for at least 10 min per day – Exercises to improve balance and to reduce risk of falls and injuries related – Those with chronic conditions for which the physical activity is therapeutic should have a planned integrating prevention and treatment

(continued)

Table 12.2 (continued)

Recommendations	Population	Goal	Prescription
Physical Activity Guidelines for Americans (Piercy et al. 2018)	All individuals ≥ 65 years	– Gain substantial health benefits	– The same amount as the WHO recommendations. Considerations for those that cannot performed de 150 min of moderate-intensity activity – Aerobic exercises: should be performed at least 3 days-week – To prevent falls and imbalance problems, balance exercises and muscle-strengthening activities should be performed at least 3 days-week for a total of 90 min, in addition to moderate-intensity aerobic exercise at least 1 h a week

an individual's vulnerability for developing increased dependency and/or death." (Morley et al. 2013). Old age and unhealthy lifestyle were associated with greater physical frailty (Gobbens et al. 2010b). The reduction in physical activity as people getting older can both predict or exacerbate frail (Liu and Fielding 2011; Fried 2016) . Thus, physical activity can be an important modifiable lifestyle factor to both preventing and treating the physical component of frailty in older adults (BGS 2014).

Several molecular mechanisms contribute to the development of frailty, such as cellular senescence, loss of telomeric structures, mitochondrial dysfunction, increase free radical production and poor capability to repair deoxyribonucleic acid (Walston et al. 2006). These mechanisms culminate in neuromuscular changes, dysfunction of the immune system and neuroendocrine dysregulation (Walston et al. 2006). The neuromuscular changes are marked by sarcopenia, i.e. skeletal muscle loss. Muscle replacement by adipose tissue (Visser et al. 2002) leads to reduced strength, decreased exercise tolerance and reduced functional capacity (Zampieri et al. 2014). Inflammatory cytokines (IL-6), bioactive hormones and preserved function of the sympathetic and central nervous system are essential to the maintenance of skeletal muscle (Ershler and Keller 2000). Physical activity improves the systems related to frailty etiology, including neuromuscular, hormonal, inflammatory, immune, hematologic and brain functions (Liu and Fielding 2011; Fried 2016)

There is evidence that physical exercise are efficacy in the treatment of frailty, being recommended by guidelines (Fairhall et al. 2011; BGS 2014; Dent et al. 2017) and committees (Morley et al. 2013). However, current health-care for frailty is mainly secondary based treatment and reactive to acute outcomes, such as falls and delirium (Turner and Clegg 2014). It is imperative that exercises should be prescribed to prevent the occurrence of frailty and pre-frailty, to reverse these statuses, and to prevent adverse outcomes that those with frailty are more predisposed for.

The benefits of physical exercises for pre-frail and frail older adults are (Theou et al. 2011; de Labra et al. 2015; BGS 2014):

- Mobility improvement;
- Strength and power enhance;
- Fatigue reduced;
- Functional capacity improvement;

- Balance control improvement;
- Diminished need of care;
- Preventing falls;
- Changes in body composition;
- Decreased likelihood of admission to a hospital or nursing home;
- Reversal of frailty.

As frailty affects negatively multiple physiological systems, a multicomponent exercise program (resistance, aerobic, balance, flexibility and functional activities training) is the most effective intervention for this population (Bray et al. 2016; Jadczak et al. 2018). Physiological adaptations occur with the practice of exercises and each type of exercise will act at specific components of frailty (Aguirre and Villareal 2015).

One of the essentials types of exercises and that must be included in any intervention for frail older adults is resistance training or strength exercises (Jadczak et al. 2018). Resistance training is fundamental for prevention and for treatment of sarcopenia (Theou et al. 2011; BGS 2014; Dent et al. 2017). There is a claim that maybe sarcopenia could be the starting point for the development of frailty, and therefore avoiding it effectively can prevent the progress of the remainder physical frailty phenotype (Xue et al. 2012). Resistance exercise promotes neuromuscular adaptations (Cadore et al. 2014), with motor performance, muscle mass and strength improvement (Liu and Fielding 2011), and thus can positive influence most of the components of the physical frailty phenotype.

The decline in strength in the older adults is explained in large part by the selective atrophy of type II muscle fibers (Aguirre and Villareal 2015). This atrophy is caused by high levels of inflammatory cytokines that have a direct catabolic effect on skeletal muscle (Aguirre and Villareal 2015). Strength training can suppress inflammatory factors, promoting anabolism and muscle protein synthesis leading to muscle hypertrophy, increase recruitment capacity, strength gain and muscle power (Cadore et al. 2014; Aguirre and Villareal 2015). To promote marked muscle strength gains, the resistance training for frail older adults should be performed 2–3 times a week, starting with high repetitions (3 sets of 12–15 repetitions) and low intensity (30–55% of 1RM) progressing to low repetitions (3 sets of 8 repetitions) and high intensity (80% of 1RM) (Cadore et al. 2014; Bray et al. 2016).

Endurance and balance training are often included within a multicomponent exercise program for frail older adults (Theou et al. 2011; Cadore et al. 2013; Dent et al. 2017).

Aerobic or endurance exercises, such as walking, stationary cycling, can change the frailty phenotype by improving the maximal oxygen uptake (VO_2 peak), increasing muscle mass, and decreasing fatigability (Liu and Fielding 2011; Aguirre and Villareal 2015). Older adults present reduction in the supply O_2 to the muscles and difficulty of the muscle to extract the O_2 (Aguirre and Villareal 2015). Aerobic training increases capillary density resulting in greater myoglobin content and greater mitochondrial biogenesis (Zampieri et al. 2014). These adaptations rise VO_{2max} and the ability of the muscle to generate energy via oxidative metabolism (Cadore et al. 2014). The endurance training should be performed 2–3 days a week starting with 5–10 min progressing to 15–30 min (Cadore et al. 2014) and with an intensity of perceived exertion of 3–4 (somewhat hard) on the Borg scale (Bray et al. 2016).

Balance exercises are important for this population as they are at higher risk of falls (Bray et al. 2016). Static and dynamic balance training can be performed with several stimuli (Bray et al. 2016), such as eyes open and closed, diminished the base of support (feet together, tandem), gait velocity, gait change directions and others. The training should be performed 2–3 days a week for 8–20 min (Bray et al. 2016).

Flexibility training or stretching exercises, although not mandatory, can be helpful within a multicomponent exercise for frail older adults, to improve range of motion (Stathokostas et al. 2012). This type of exercise can be performed integrated to the other trainings or separately as part of the cool-down for 7–10 min in 2–3 days a week (Bray et al. 2016).

Exercises simulating activities of daily living, such as star climbing, changing between positions, are important to functional independence (Bray et al. 2016; Liu et al. 2016). It seems that older adults do not fully translate physiological gains from regular exercise (strength, flexibility) to improve in their performance in daily activities (Liu et al. 2016), i.e. they could have quadriceps strength but cannot raise from a chair. Exercises task oriented might be ideal to prevent disability and frailty in older adults.

Regardless of the type of exercise there is evidence that physical exercise interventions for frail older adults improve normal gait speed (mean difference: 0.07 m/s; 95% CI: 0.04–0.09), fast gait speed (mean difference: 0.08 m/s; 95% CI: 0.02–0.14), the Short Physical Performance Battery (mean difference: 2.18; 95% CI: 1.56–2.80) and the Chair Raise test (mean difference: 2.35 s; 95% CI: 0.35–4.35) comparing to inactive control. No between groups differences were found for general physical function scales, mobility (Timed Up and Go), balance tests (tandem, one leg stance) and independency in daily activities (Giné-Garriga et al. 2014). For mild or pre-frail older adults, the evidence is scarce, due to small samples, insufficient and not high-quality trials (Frost et al. 2017). A quantitative synthesis with 5 trials revealed that exercises interventions for pre-frail older adults had superior benefits than control in performance-based functioning (mean difference: 0.37; 95% CI: 0.07–0.68), balance (mean difference: 0.33; 95% CI: 0.08–0.57) and muscle strength (mean difference: 0.44; 95% CI: 0.11–0.77). No effects were found on self-reported functioning, gait speed and Timed Up and Go (Frost et al. 2017). An umbrella review (Jadczak et al. 2018) summarized the evidence (seven systematic reviews—58 randomized control trials) regarding effectiveness of exercises interventions to improve physical function in frail older people. The authors founded that there is an overall increase in muscle strength (n = 5 trials increase vs. n = 2 trials no effects), gait speed (n = 7 trials increase vs. n = 3 trials effects), balance (n = 8 trials increase vs. n = 1 trials no effects) and physical performance (n = 16 trials increase vs. n = 1 trials no effects) with a multicomponent training. The physical outcome, mobility, had no overall effect in frail older adults (n = 9 trials increase vs. n = 10 trials no effects) (Jadczak et al. 2018).

Although there is evidence that physical exercises are benefic to frail older adults, still it is unclear the best type, intensity and duration (Giné-Garriga et al. 2014; de Labra et al. 2015; Dent et al. 2017; Puts et al. 2017; Jadczak et al. 2018). Some prescriptions go from 3 times a week for 45 of up to 60 min per session for pre-frail older adults (Bray et al. 2016) and 2–3 times a week for 30 of up to 45–60 min, for frail older adults (Theou et al. 2011; Cadore et al. 2013; Bray et al. 2016; Jadczak et al. 2018). The physical practice should start with more accessible and safe exercises (Liu and Fielding 2011; Bray et al. 2016), such as chair exercises, non-weight bearing activities, walking and elastic band exercises. The exercises should progressively intensify on the individuals' capability and performance (Puts et al. 2017). The exercise progression is mandatory to promote gains in physiological function and must be at the level of the activities of daily living performance to ensure functional independence (Bray et al. 2016). For those severely frail it is advised to perform exercises with the orientation of a rehabilitation professional (Liu and Fielding 2011). For better adherence the physical program should be supervised and individually tailored to the frail older adult (Dent et al. 2017). There is a dissipation of the effect once frail individuals discontinue the practice of exercises (Giné-Garriga et al. 2014). Therefore, for long term benefits, it is central to continue practicing exercises and stimulating older adults to be more physically active and reduce sedentary time (Dent et al. 2017).

Is important to highlight that there is no contraindication to frail older adults be engaged in physical activities (Aguirre and Villareal 2015) and in physical rehabilitation (Gustavson et al. 2017). Trials with frail older adults revealed very low occurrence of adverse effects during the practice of exercises program (Liu and Fielding 2011; Giné-Garriga et al. 2014; Puts et al. 2017). A systematic review with meta-analysis found no difference between inactive control group and experimental group practicing exercises regarding the occurrence of adverse effects such as fractures, tendinitis, muscular soreness, back pain, musculoskeletal injures and falls in frail older adults (Giné-Garriga et al. 2014). Thus, precautions with the practice of physical exercises for frailty should be the same as the older population in general.

12.4 Physical Exercise for Cardiovascular Disease

As people become older, the cardiovascular system undergoes structural and functional changes that compromise cardiac reserve, predisposing for cardiovascular disorders (CVD) and decreasing physical activity capacity (Roh et al. 2016; Jakovljevic 2018). One of the most important structural changes in the cardiovascular system is a progressive loss of myocytes, i.e. the cardiac muscle cells. Consequently, there are mild hypertrophy of the cardiac muscle and a decreased in the sensitivity to sympathetic stimuli, which will compromise myocardial contractility and the ability to pump blood (Lakatta 2002; Lakatta and Levy 2003). Regarding vascular changes, collagen decrease, calcium deposition and fragmentation of the elastic fibers are observed with aging, culminating in enlarged arteries and thicker and stiffer walls (Lakatta 2002; Jakovljevic 2018). Thus, it is common that older people face cardiovascular pathophysiological conditions such as left ventricular hypertrophy, chronic heart failure, atrial fibrillation and atherosclerosis (Lakatta and Levy 2003; Jakovljevic 2018).

CVD's are the leading contributors to disease burden in older people, being the main cause of death, causing considerable disability and reducing well-being (Li and Siegrist 2012). In 2010, CVD were responsible for 30% of total DALYs (disability-adjusted life years), being the most frequent cause the ischemic heart disease (Prince et al. 2015). The control of CVD should happen using preventive measures and be treat in the primary care level, i.e. before the disease seriously affect a person (Buttar et al. 2005). However, when the CVD is installed, cardiac rehabilitation will provide secondary prevention in order to stabilize, slow or reverse disease progression, and, also to preserve patient functional capacity to perform daily activities (Price et al. 2016).

There is evidence that CVD is preventable and treatable by lifestyle changes (Buttar et al. 2005). One of the most important modifiable risk factors for CVD is physical inactivity. Physical activity and exercise can attenuate age-related cardiovascular changes by improving the cardiovascular system, cardiac function and metabolism (Jakovljevic 2018) . Physical exercise has a protective effect on CVD because it acts in the deceleration of the atherosclerotic process (improve endothelial function and lipid profile; and decrease inflammation markers and thrombosis) and controlling risk factors, such as hypertension, diabetes, and obesity (decrease insulin and vascular resistance and diminish sympathetic activity) (Cheng et al. 2013). In general, the exercise prescriptions for patients with CVD should always be individualized, especially for older adults that have other associated comorbidities (Pedersen and Saltin 2006). The practice of physical exercises by older people with CVD appears to be safe and should be done regularly (NHFA 2006). Bellow we present the effects of exercises in the cardiovascular system and for the most common CVD conditions in older adults.

12.4.1 Effect of Exercise on Blood Coagulation and Fibrinolysis

Blood coagulation and fibrinolysis are physiological factors that influence the development of blood clots and its breakdown within vessels (Buttar et al. 2005). Increased fibrinogen concentrations and platelet aggregation factors rise the risk of ischemic cardiovascular events, e.g. heart attack and stroke (Buttar et al. 2005).

Long-term aerobic exercise leads to decreased coagulation potential (Womack et al. 2003) and increased fibrinolytic potential (Li et al. 2007).

12.4.2 Effect of Exercise on Vascular Remodeling

Vascular endothelial cells produce nitric oxide that has vasodilatory function (Taddei et al. 2000). With aging the action of nitric oxide is reduced (Taddei et al. 2000). However, moderate aerobic exercise significantly increases the plasma concentration of this vasodilator (Maeda et al. 2004). Thus, the exercise leads to increased arterial lumen resulting in reduced resistance to blood flow and maximizes tissue perfusion. Reduced resistance decreases the risk of CVD (i.e. hypertension) and increases blood flow in areas that may have undergone ischemia (Buttar et al. 2005).

12.4.3 Effect of Exercise on Blood Lipid Profiles

There is a direct relationship between chronically elevated cholesterol levels and coronary heart disease. Evidence shows that exercise has beneficial effects in individuals with dyslipidemia, since they appear to reduce total cholesterol levels (Buttar et al. 2005) . Physical exercise causes the muscle to increase lipid consumption as a source of energy. This process increases the activity of lipoprotein lipase that coincides with increase in HDL cholesterol (Earnest et al. 2013). HDL cholesterol acts by collecting excess LDL (responsible for forming atheromatous plaques) that has been deposited in vascular tissue reducing total cholesterol levels (Ohashi et al. 2005).

12.4.4 Effect of Exercise on Blood Pressure and Hypertension

Blood pressure is determined by cardiac output and vascular resistance. Prolonged practice of aerobic exercise leads to a reduction in vascular resistance and consequent decrease in blood pressure (Pescatello et al. 2004). These adaptations are due to sympathetic nervous system-mediated increase in vessel diameter and the humoral renin-angiotensin system (Cheng et al. 2013). For those with hypertension it is recommended the practice of aerobic exercises of moderate intensity (40–60% VO_2) at least 30 min per day (Pescatello et al. 2004; Pedersen and Saltin 2006).

12.4.5 Coronary Heart Disease

For coronary heart disease, the European Society of Cardiology recommends aerobic physical exercises of moderate intensity (Giannuzzi et al. 2003). Low-risk patients should perform 30–60 min per week of aerobic exercise with 55–70% of the maximum workload. For moderate to high-risk patients, exercise prescription is similar, but should start with a maximum work load of less than 50%. Resistance exercise should last at least 1 h per week with intensity of 10–15 repetitions per set (Piepoli et al. 2010).

12.4.6 Chronic Heart Failure

For those with chronic heart failure, aerobic training should be performed with intensity and duration gradually increasing (Pedersen and Saltin 2006). During initial stage, intensity should be kept at a low level (40–50% of peak VO_2), increasing the duration from 15 to 30 min, 2 to 3 days a week according to the patient perceived symptoms and clinical status. After the acute phase, a gradual increase in intensity (50, 60, 70–80% of peak VO_2) should be performed (NHFA 2006; Piepoli et al. 2010).

To reduce cardiovascular mortality, healthy individuals of all ages should perform moderate-intensity aerobic physical activity of at least 30 min in most days of the week with weekly energy expenditure of about 1000 kcal (Giannuzzi et al. 2003). For those with CVD the recommendation is to perform exercises through cardiac rehabilitation (Giannuzzi et al. 2003; NHFA 2006;

Piepoli et al. 2010). Cardiac rehabilitation is a multidisciplinary intervention that includes health education, physical activity and stress management to patients with heart diseases or cardiac procedures, such as post-myocardial infarction, post-coronary artery by-pass grafting, heart failure and others (Giannuzzi et al. 2003; Cacciatore et al. 2016). Physical rehabilitation should be implemented in accordance with the risk assessment criteria to exercises and adapted to the different CVD patterns (Cacciatore et al. 2016).

It is a consensus from guidelines and societies recommendations-statements that the aerobic endurance training is the foundation for cardiac rehabilitation (Price et al. 2016). However, the intensity and duration prescription varied broadly, from 40 to 80% of VO_2, 40–85% of Heart Rate Reserve, 1–5 days a week and 15–60 min (Price et al. 2016). The practice of strengthening exercises has been recommended in association with aerobic exercises (Piepoli et al. 2010). Resistance load prescription varies from 30 to 80% of 1RM and on the individual's level of fatigue (Price et al. 2016). Regarding flexibility exercises, they are not routinely specified as a component of cardiac rehabilitation because of the paucity of evidence regarding the benefits to this population (Price et al. 2016).

The performance of older adults with CVD during physical exercises should be monitoring by parameters, such as heart rate, Borg Rating of Perceived Exertion Scale, blood pressure, breathlessness, fatigue, chest pain and lightheadedness, in order to adapt the treatment, to achieve better results and to avoid adverse effects (Price et al. 2016).

Although, there is evidence of the protective role of physical exercise on CVD, the exact dose-response (type, intensity and duration) is still uncertain, even further for older adult population (Cheng et al. 2013). Thus, rehabilitation programs for CVD vary in their frequency and intensity (Price et al. 2016). A metanalysis (Li and Siegrist 2012) revealed that high level of leisure time physical activity reduces the risk of CVD in 24% (men) to 27% (women) compared to those with low level, while moderate intensity decreases the risk 18% (women) to 20% (men). Regarding occupational physical activity a protective effect was found for moderate level of 11% (men) to 17% (women), whereas high physical activity at work fails to show stronger protective effect against CVD (Li and Siegrist 2012). Thus, there is a dose-response relationship between physical activity and CVD (Li and Siegrist 2012). It seems that moderate exercise is the desirable activity level for increase benefits in patients with CVD (Buttar et al. 2005). This agrees with the recommendations of The National Heart Foundation of Australia in which people with stable CVD should be engaged in 30 min or more of moderate-intensity physical activity on most days of a week for health benefits and those with advanced CVD may have to practice for a lesser amount (NHFA 2006).

Regardless of all benefits, physical exercises should be prescribed with some caution on older adults with CVD (Viña et al. 2016). Thus, without a professional advice even low-intensity exercises may not be advisable for patients with chronic heart failure or had an acute heart attack (Buttar et al. 2005). There are some CVD that are considered contraindications for physical exercises, such as unstable angina, severe aortic stenosis, uncontrolled cardiac failure, pericarditis, myocarditis, endocarditis, fever and severe hypertension (NHFA 2006). It is also advised that during exercises Valsalva maneuvers should be avoided, especially in patients with high blood pressure (Viña et al. 2016). Although there are some contraindications, this should not constrain to prescribe it, as exercises through cardiac rehabilitation demonstrated to be feasible, safe and efficacy to older people (Fattirolli and Pratesi 2015).

Despite the benefits and recommendations above mentioned of regular physical exercises for patients with CVD, it is important that the exercise routine integrates a treatment with other measures (nutrition, medication, professional orientation) to achieve better results.

12.5 Physical Exercise for Frailty and Cardiovascular Disease-Working Together

The previous sections of this chapter have showed the characteristics of the frailty syndrome and the CVD and its relationship to physical activity and exercises separately. However, as it was possible to notice, these conditions share many biological aspects, symptoms and adverse effects. Thus, when present concurrently the older adult is exposed to a worse prognosis and is at high risk for functional disability (Fattirolli and Pratesi 2015). The importance to identify older adults with both conditions is to anticipate major cardiac events (Singh et al. 2008), prevent hospitalizations, and avoid physical deconditioning. Therefore, the practice of physical exercises, through physical rehabilitation, is mandatory for older adults that presents these conditions.

Before of a clearly clinical diagnosis of CVD, frail older adults already exhibit subclinical cardiovascular derangements (Afilalo et al. 2014). A systematic review found that in older adults, CVD increases 2.7–4.1 the chance for prevalent frailty and 1.5 for incident frailty (those not frail at baseline) (Afilalo et al. 2009). Alterations in inflammatory and immune cells encountered in both conditions affects the arterial wall and promote atherosclerosis (Afilalo et al. 2014).

Older adults represent more than one third of those referred to cardiac rehabilitation and a substantial proportion are also frailty (Fattirolli and Pratesi 2015; Vigorito et al. 2017). Cardiac rehabilitation presents benefits for older adults with both conditions. Particularly, improvements with exercises through cardiac rehabilitation are observed in frailty older adults that needs cardiac surgery (Afilalo et al. 2014). In these cases, to facilitate recovery, rehabilitation should be pre- and post-cardiac procedure. Unfortunately, cardiovascular rehabilitation for older adults has lower referral rate and is underused (Fattirolli and Pratesi 2015; Flint et al. 2018). One study (Flint et al. 2018) regarding older adults after one month of acute myocardial infarction and gait speed (a mark of physical frailty) revealed that compared to those with normal gait speed, older adults with slow gait speed were less likely to be referred to cardiac rehabilitation (55.7% vs. 68.9%) and were less likely to participate in it (27.1% vs. 40.1%). At one-year follow-up slow gait speed and lack of participation on cardiac rehabilitation were associated with higher rates of death or disability (Flint et al. 2018).

A good physical exercise program should consider the typical physiologic alterations that occurs in older adults adding vulnerability of the frail syndrome and the standard cardiac limitations in those with CVD. Both aerobic capacity and muscle strength is markedly reduced in these conditions. In the Longitudinal Aging Study Amsterdam (LASA) (Kleipool et al. 2018), it was found that excepting for the weight loss, all other four components of the physical frailty phenotype were statistical higher in older adults with CVD comparing with those without CDV. The component with higher prevalence between those with CVD was weak grip strength (56%) (Kleipool et al. 2018).

A multicomponent program with endure and strength training is desirable to improve the neurohormonal, inflammatory and metabolic parameters related to frailty and CVD (Vigorito et al. 2017). The exercise prescription should be influenced by the older adult risk profile regarding these conditions (Cacciatore et al. 2016). Despite the evidence of the benefits of exercises in both conditions isolated (Giannuzzi et al. 2003; de Labra et al. 2015; Pedersen and Saltin 2006; Li and Siegrist 2012; Cadore et al. 2013; Frost et al. 2017; Jadczak et al. 2018), there is need to future studies to investigate the effects of physical exercises on those that share frailty and CVD. The Cardiac Rehabilitation Section of the European Association of Preventive Cardiology (EAPC) proposed a call to action to cardiac rehabilitation for older adults with CVD and frailty (Vigorito et al. 2017). First recommendation is for professionals in the cardiac rehabilitation setting to use instruments to recognize and evaluate frailty. Then, prescribe exercise-based cardiac rehabilitation through tailored interventions for these conditions.

For those frail older adults with CVD at high risk or cannot go to an outpatient clinic, home-based exercises are an option. Also, it is important to give instructions to caregivers and family to stimulate them to be more active during daily activities reducing sedentary behavior. For long term results it is important for those frail older adults with CVD to change lifestyle including better eating habits, control weight, practice regularly physical exercises and be more active. All these will help in the controlling of such conditions.

Acknowledgments We thank Brendon Stubbs for improving the use of English in this Chapter.

References

ACSM-American College of Sports Medicine, Chodzko-Zajko WJ, Proctor DN, Fiatarone Singh MA, Minson CT, Nigg CR et al (2009) American College of Sports Medicine position stand. Exercise and physical activity for older adults. Med Sci Sports Exerc 41(7):1510–1530. https://doi.org/10.1249/mss.0b013e3181a0c95c

Afilalo J, Karunananthan S, Eisenberg MJ, Alexander KP, Bergman H (2009) Role of frailty in patients with cardiovascular disease. Am J Cardiol 103(11):1616–1621. https://doi.org/10.1016/j.amjcard.2009.01.375

Afilalo J, Alexander KP, Mack MJ, Maurer MS, Green P, Allen LA et al (2014) Frailty assessment in the cardiovascular care of older adults. J Am Coll Cardiol 63 (8):747–762. https://doi.org/10.1016/j.jacc.2013.09.070

Aguirre LE, Villareal DT (2015) Physical exercise as therapy for frailty. Nestle Nutr Inst Workshop Ser 83:83–92. https://doi.org/10.1159/000382065

BGS-British Geriatrics Society (2014) Fit for Frailty—consensus best practice guidance for the care of older people living in community and outpatient settings—a report from the British Geriatrics Society. https://www.bgs.org.uk/sites/default/files/content/resources/files/2018-05-23/fff_full.pdf. Accessed 10 Dec 2018

Bray NW, Smart RR, Jakobi JM, Jones GR (2016) Exercise prescription to reverse frailty. Appl Physiol Nutr Metab 41(10):1112–1116

Buttar HS, Li T, Ravi N (2005) Prevention of cardiovascular diseases: role of exercise, dietary interventions, obesity and smoking cessation. Exp Clin Cardiol 10 (4):229–249

Cacciatore F, Ferrara N, Mezzani A, Maiello C, Amarelli C, Curcio F et al (2016) Cardiac rehabilitation in the elderly patients. Sports Med Rehabil J 1 (2):1006

Cadore EL, Rodriguez-Manas L, Sinclair A, Izquierdo M (2013) Effects of different exercise interventions on risk of falls, gait ability, and balance in physically frail older adults: a systematic review. Rejuvenation Res 16 (2):105–114. https://doi.org/10.1089/rej.2012.1397

Cadore EL, Pinto RS, Bottaro M, Izquierdo M (2014) Strength and endurance training prescription in healthy and frail elderly. Aging Dis 5(3):183–195. https://doi.org/10.14336/AD.2014.0500183

Caspersen CJ, Powell KE, Christenson GM (1985) Physical activity, exercise, and physical fitness: definitions and distinctions for health-related research. Public Health Rep 100(2):126–131

Cheng S-J, Yu H-K, Chen Y-C, Chen C-Y, Lien W-C, Yang P-Y et al (2013) Physical activity and risk of cardiovascular disease among older adults. Int J Gerontol 7:133–136

Daskalopoulou C, Stubbs B, Kralj C, Koukounari A, Prince M, Prina AM (2017) Physical activity and healthy ageing: A systematic review and meta-analysis of longitudinal cohort studies. Ageing Res Rev 38:6–17. https://doi.org/10.1016/j.arr.2017.06.003

Dent E, Lien C, Lim WS, Wong WC, Wong CH, Ng TP et al (2017) The Asia-Pacific clinical practice guidelines for the management of frailty. J Am Med Dir Assoc 18(7):564–575. https://doi.org/10.1016/j.jamda.2017.04.018

Earnest CP, Artero EG, Sui X, Church TS, Blair SN (2013) Maximal estimated cardiorespiratory fitness, cardiometabolic risk factors, and metabolic syndrome in the aerobics center longitudinal study. Mayo Clin Proc 88(3):259–570

Elsawy B, Higgins KE (2010) Physical activity guidelines for older adults. Am Fam Phys 81(1):55–59

Ershler WB, Keller ET (2000) Age-associated increased interleukin-6 gene expression, late life diseases, and frailty. Annu Rev Med 51:245–270

Fairhall N, Langron C, Sherrington C, Lord SR, Kurrle SE, Lockwood K et al (2011) Treating frailty: a practical guide. BMC Med 9:83. https://doi.org/10.1186/1741-7015-9-83

Fattirolli F, Pratesi A (2015) Cardiovascular prevention and rehabilitation in the elderly: evidence for cardiac rehabilitation after myocardial infarction or chronic heart failure. Monaldi Arch Chest Dis 84:731

Flint K, Kennedy K, Arnold SV, Dodson JA, Cresci S, Alexander KP (2018) Slow gait speed and cardiac rehabilitation participation in older adults after acute myocardial infarction. J Am Heart Assoc 7(5): e008296. https://doi.org/10.1161/JAHA.117.008296

Fried LP, Tangen CM, Walston J, Newman AB, Hirsch C, Gottdiener J et al (2001) Frailty in older adults: evidence for a phenotype. J Gerontol A Biol Sci Med Sci 56(3):M146–M156

Fried LP (2016) Interventions for human frailty: physical activity as a model. Cold Spring Harb Perspect Med. 6:a025916

Frost R, Belk C, Jovicic A, RicciardiF, Kharicha K, Gardner B et al (2017) Health promotion interventions for community-dwelling older people with mild or pre-frailty: a systematic review and meta-analysis. BMC Geriatr 17(1):157. https://doi.org/10.1186/s12877-017-0547-8

García-Peña C, Ávila-Funes JA, Dent E, Gutiérrez-Robledo L, Pérez-Zepeda M (2016) Frailty prevalence and associated factors in the Mexican health and aging study: a comparison of the frailty index and the phenotype. Exp Gerontol 79:55–60

Giannuzzi P, Mezzani A, Saner H, Bjornstad H, Fioretti P, Mendes M et al (2003) Physical activity for primary and secondary prevention. Position paper of the working group on cardiac rehabilitation and exercise physiology of the European Society of Cardiology. Eur J Cardiovasc Prev Rehabil 10:319–327

Giné-Garriga M, Roqué-Fíguls M, Coll-Planas L, Sitjà-Rabert M, Salvà A (2014) Physical exercise interventions for improving performance-based measures of physical function in community-dwelling, frail older adults: a systematic review and meta-analysis. Arch Phys Med Rehabil 95(4):753–769. https://doi.org/10.1016/j.apmr.2013.11.007

Gobbens RJJ, Luijkx KG, Wijnen-Sponselee MT, Schols JMGA (2010a) In search of an integral conceptual definition of frailty: opinions of experts. J Am Med Dir Assoc 11:338–343

Gobbens RJ, van Assen MA, Luijkx KG, Wijnen-Sponselee MT, Schols JM (2010b) Determinants of frailty. J Am Med Dir Assoc 11(5):356–364. https://doi.org/10.1016/j.jamda.2009.11.008

González K, Fuentes J, Márquez JL (2017) Physical inactivity, sedentary behavior and chronic diseases. Korean J Fam Med. 38(3):111–115. https://doi.org/10.4082/kjfm.2017.38.3.111

Gustavson AM, Falvey JR, Jankowski CM, Stevens-Lapsley JE (2017) Public health impact of frailty: role of physical therapists. J Frailty Aging 6(1):2–5. https://doi.org/10.14283/jfa.2017.1

Jadczak AD, Makwana N, Luscombe-Marsh N, Visvanathan R, Schultz TJ (2018) Effectiveness of exercise interventions on physical function in community-dwelling frail older people. JBI Database Syst Rev Implement Rep 16(3):752–775. https://doi.org/10.11124/jbisrir-2017-003551

Jakovljevic DG (2018) Physical activity and cardiovascular aging: physiological and molecular insights. Exp Gerontol 109:67–74. https://doi.org/10.1016/j.exger.2017.05.016

Kleipool EE, Hoogendijk EO, Trappenburg MC, Handoko ML, Huisman M, Peters MJ et al (2018) Frailty in older adults with cardiovascular disease: cause, effect or both? Aging Dis 9(3):489–497. https://doi.org/10.14336/AD.2017.1125

de Labra C, Guimaraes-Pinheiro C, Maseda A, Lorenzo T, Millán-Calenti JC (2015) Effects of physical exercise interventions in frail older adults: a systematic review of randomized controlled trials. BMC Geriatr 15:154. https://doi.org/10.1186/s12877-015-0155-4

Lakatta EG (2002) Age-associated cardiovascular changes in health: impact on cardiovascular disease in older persons. Heart Fail Rev 7(1): 29–49

Lakatta EG, Levy D (2003) Arterial and cardiac aging: major shareholders in cardiovascular disease enterprises: part II: the aging heart in health: links to heart disease. Circulation 107(2):346–354

Li J, Siegrist J (2012) Physical activity and risk of cardiovascular disease: a meta-analysis of prospective cohort studies. Int J Environ Res Public Health. 9:391–407. https://doi.org/10.3390/ijerph9020391

Li N, He S, Blombäck M, Hjemdahl P (2007) Platelet activity, coagulation, and fibrinolysis during exercise in healthy males: effects of thrombin inhibition by argatroban and enoxaparin. Arterioscler Thrombos Vasc Biol 27(2):407–413

Liu CK, Fielding RA (2011) Exercise as an intervention for frailty. Clin Geriatr Med 27(1):101–110

Liu CJ, Jones LY, Formyduval ARM, Clark DO (2016) Task-oriented exercise to reduce activities of daily living disability in vulnerable older adults: a feasibility study of the 3-step workout for life. J Aging Phys Act 24 (3):384–392

Maeda S, Tanabe T, Otsuki T, Sugawara J, Iemitsu M, Miyauchi T, Matsuda M (2004) Moderate regular exercise increases basal production of nitric oxide in elderly women. Hypertens Res 27(12):947–953

Matthews CE, Chen KY, Freedson PS, Buchowski MS, Beech BM, Pate RR et al (2008) Amount of time spent in sedentary behaviors in the United States, 2003–2004. Am J Epidemiol 167(7):875–881. https://doi.org/10.1093/aje/kwm390

Morley JE, Vellas B, van Kan GA, Anker SD, Bauer JM, Bernabei R et al (2013) Frailty consensus: a call to action. J Am Med Dir Assoc 14(6):392–397

Nadruz W, Kitzman D, Windham BG, Kucharska-Newton A, Butler K, Palta P et al (2017) Cardiovascular dysfunction and frailty among older adults in the community: the ARIC study. J Gerontol A Biol Sci Med Sci 72(7):958–964

Nelson ME, Rejeski WJ, Blair SN, Duncan PW, Judge JO, King AC, Macera CA, Castaneda-Sceppa C (2007) Physical activity and public health in older adults: recommendation from the American College of Sports Medicine and the American Heart Association. Med Sci Sports Exerc 39(8):1435–1445

NHFA-National Heart Foundation of Australia (2006) Physical activity in patients with cardiovascular disease: management algorithm and information for general practice. Melbourne: National Heart Foundation of Australia. https://www.heartfoundation.org.au/images/uploads/publications/physical-activity-in-patients-with-cvd-management-algorithm.pdf. Accessed 08 Jan 2019

Ohashi R, Mu H, Wang X, Yao Q, Chen C (2005) Reverse cholesterol transport and cholesterol efflux in atherosclerosis. QJM 98(12):845–856

Pedersen BK, Saltin B (2006) Evidence for prescribing exercise as therapy in chronic disease. Scand J Med Sci Sports 16(Suppl 1):3–63

Perracini MR, Franco MRC, Ricci NA, Blake C (2017) Physical activity in older people: case studies of how to make change happen. Best Pract Res Clin Rheumatol 31 (2):260–274. https://doi.org/10.1016/j.berh.2017.08.007

Pescatello LS, Franklin BA, Fagard R, Farquhar WB, Kelley GA, Ray CA (2004) Exercise and hypertension. Med Sci Sports Exerc 36(3):533–553

Piepoli MF, Corra U, Benzer W, Bjarnason-Wehrens B, Dendale P, Gaita D, Schmid JP (2010) Secondary prevention through cardiac rehabilitation: from knowledge to implementation. A position paper from the Cardiac Rehabilitation Section of the European Association of Cardiovascular Prevention and Rehabilitation. Euro J Cardiovasc Prev Rehabil 17(1):1–17

Piercy KL, Troiano RP, Ballard RM, Carlson SA, Fulton JE, Galuska DA (2018) The physical activity guidelines for Americans. JAMA 320(19):2020–2028. https://doi.org/10.1001/jama.2018.14854

Price KJ, Gordon BA, Bird SR, Benson AC (2016) A review of guidelines for cardiac rehabilitation exercise programmes: is there an international consensus? Eur J Prev Cardiol 23(16):1715–1733

Prince MJ, Wu F, Guo Y, Gutierrez Robledo LM, O'Donnell M, Sullivan R et al (2015) The burden of disease in older people and implications for health policy and practice. Lancet 385(9967):549–562. https://doi.org/10.1016/S0140-6736(14)61347-7

Puts MTE, Toubasi S, Andrew MK, Ashe MC, Ploeg J, Atkinson E et al (2017) Interventions to prevent or reduce the level of frailty in community-dwelling older adults: a scoping review of the literature and international policies. Age Ageing 46(3):383–392

Roh J, Rhee J, Chaudhari V, Rosenzweig A (2016) The role of exercise in cardiac aging: from physiology to molecular mechanisms. Circ Res 118(2):279–295. https://doi.org/10.1161/CIRCRESAHA.115.305250

SBRN-Sedentary Behavior Research Network (2012) Letter to the Editor: Standardized use of the terms "sedentary" and "sedentary behaviours". Appl Physiol Nutr Metab 37(3):540–542

Singh M, Alexander K, Roger VL, Rihal CS, Whitson HE, Lerman A et al (2008) Frailty and its potential relevance to cardiovascular care. Mayo Clin Proc 83 (10):1146–1153

Sparling PB, Howard BJ, Dunstan DW, Owen N (2015) Recommendations for physical activity in older adults. BMJ 350:h100. https://doi.org/10.1136/bmj.h100

Stathokostas L, Little R, Vandervoort AA, Paterson DH (2012) Flexibility training and functional ability in older adults: a systematic review. J Aging Res 2012:306818. https://doi.org/10.1155/2012/306818

Taddei S, Galetta F, Virdis A, Ghiadoni L, Salvetti G, Franzoni F et al (2000) Physical activity prevents age-related impairment in nitric oxide availability in elderly athletes. Circulation 101:2896–2901

Theou O, Stathokostas L, Roland KP, Jakobi JM, Patterson C, Vandervoort AA et al (2011) The effectiveness of exercise interventions for the management of frailty: a systematic review. J Aging Res 569194. https://doi.org/10.4061/2011/569194

Turner G, Clegg A (2014) Best practice guidelines for the management of frailty: a British Geriatrics Society, age UK and Royal College of General Practitioners report. Age Ageing 43:744–747. https://doi.org/10.1093/ageing/afu138

Tremblay MS, Aubert S, Barnes JD, Saunders TJ, Carson V, Latimer-Cheung AE et al (2017) Sedentary Behavior Research Network (SBRN): terminology consensus project process and outcome. Int J Behav Nutr Phys Act. 14(1):75

Vigorito C, Abreu A, Ambrosetti M, Belardinelli R, Corrà U, Cupples M et al (2017) Frailty and cardiac rehabilitation: a call to action from the EAPC Cardiac Rehabilitation Section. Eur J Prev Cardiol 24(6):577–590. https://doi.org/10.1177/2047487316682579

Viña J, Rodriguez-Mañas L, Salvador-Pascual A, Tarazona-Santabalbina FJ, Gomez-Cabrera MC (2016) Exercise: the lifelong supplement for healthy ageing and slowing down the onset of frailty. J Physiol 594(8):1989–1999. https://doi.org/10.1113/JP270536

Visser M, Kritchevsky SB, Goodpaster BH, Newman AB, Nevitt M, Stamm E et al (2002) Leg muscle mass and composition in relation to lower extremity performance in men and women aged 70 to 79: the Health, Aging and Body Composition Study. J Am Geriatr Soc 50:897–904

Walston J, Hadley EC, Ferrucci L, Guralnik JM, Newman AB, Studenski SA et al (2006) Research agenda for frailty in older adults: toward a better understanding of physiology and etiology: summary from the American Geriatrics Society/National Institute on Aging Research Conference on Frailty in Older Adults. J Am Geriatr Soc 54(6):991–1001

WHO World Health Organization (2010) WHO Global recommendations on physical activity for health. Geneva: World Health Organization. https://www.who.int/dietphysicalactivity/global-PA-recs-2010.pdf. Accessed 15 Nov 2018

Womack CJ, Nagelkirk PR, Coughlin AM (2003) Exercise-induced changes in coagulation and fibrinolysis in healthy populations and patients with cardiovascular disease. Sports Med 33(11):795–807

Xue QL, Bandeen-Roche K, Mielenz TJ, Seplaki CL, Szanton SL, Thorpe RJ et al (2012) Patterns of 12-year change in physical activity levels in community-dwelling older women: can modest levels of physical activity help older women live longer? Am J Epidemiol 176(6):534–543

Zampieri S, Pietrangelo L, Loefler S, Fruhmann H, Vogelauer M, Burggraf S et al (2014) Lifelong physical exercise delays age-associated skeletal muscle decline. J Gerontol A-Biol. 70(2):163–173

13 Cardiac Rehabilitation for Frail Older People

Amanda K. Buttery

Abstract

Comprehensive cardiac rehabilitation programmes include multifactorial components to optimise cardiovascular risk reduction, promote healthy behaviours and an active lifestyle, reduce disability and improve health and wellbeing. There is compelling evidence that older people with certain cardiovascular conditions, such as heart failure, can benefit both physically and mentally from cardiac rehabilitation. This chapter discusses the evolution of cardiac rehabilitation, frailty assessment in cardiac rehabilitation and guideline recommendations in the context of ageing populations. Contemporary cardiac rehabilitation service models are presented along with potential solutions to meeting older people's preferences and improving access to effective treatment for those with frailty. Innovations in catheter-based surgical interventions mean that more people with frailty are undergoing cardiovascular surgery than ever before. Although traditionally, cardiac rehabilitation has been associated with secondary prevention after cardiac diagnoses, events and interventions, new models of preconditioning rehabilitation or 'prehab' are being offered to frail older people before surgery to improve functional outcomes and reduce hospital stay. Individual tailoring of cardiac rehabilitation programme components is a cornerstone of high-quality care. Importantly, participation in core components, such as exercise and nutritional interventions, can impact on both cardiac vascular disease and frailty, providing the potential to change the trajectory of both conditions.

Keywords

Cardiac rehabilitation · Exercise · Physical activity · Cardiovascular diseases · Secondary prevention · Elderly · Frailty · Heart failure · Health services

13.1 Introduction

Despite rapid advances in treatments for cardiovascular diseases over the last 20 years, many older patients receiving medical treatment still experience problems of unrelieved symptoms. This symptomatic burden results in disability, poor quality of life and poor prognosis, with levels of morbidity and mortality for conditions such as heart failure worse than for many forms of cancer (Stewart et al. 2001).

Rehabilitation involving exercise can offer important improvements in physical function and

A. K. Buttery (✉)
Faculty of Life Sciences and Medicine,
King's College London, London, UK
e-mail: amanda.buttery@kcl.ac.uk

N. Veronese (ed.), *Frailty and Cardiovascular Diseases*, Advances in Experimental Medicine and Biology 1216, https://doi.org/10.1007/978-3-030-33330-0_13

quality of life for symptomatic patients with mildly and severely compromised cardiovascular function (Davies et al. 2010). However, the potential for considerable health gains for many older people remains unfulfilled, despite guideline recommendations for participation. Additionally, patient populations are changing, with demographic changes and innovations in catheter-based surgical interventions resulting in more people with frailty undergoing cardiovascular surgery than ever before. This change in the patient population means that cardiac rehabilitation interventions need to be underpinned by research evidence from contemporary populations. This chapter briefly describes the evolution of cardiac rehabilitation, before discussing aspects of current service models and evidence-based guidelines, and finally exploring research gaps and key areas for policy and practice of cardiac rehabilitation for frail older adults.

13.2 The Evolution of Cardiac Rehabilitation

As long ago as 1772, the physician William Heberden recognised the benefits of exercise for patients with cardiac conditions when he described that a course of sawing wood nearly 'cured' a patient with angina (Heberden 1802). Unfortunately, these early insights into the benefits of exercise on the cardiovascular system were lost, and the first half of the 1900s were characterised as a time of prescribed bed rest for many heart conditions (Dock 1944; West 2004). It was not until the 1950s and 1960s that studies of sitting out of bed to aid recovery in hospital (Levine and Lown 1952) and outpatient exercise for people with cardiac conditions, caught the interest of researchers and what we now know as cardiac rehabilitation began to develop (West 2004). Around this time the World Health Organisation (WHO) provided an early definition of cardiac rehabilitation (World Health Organisation 1964), emphasising recovery and return to previous health, stating cardiac rehabilitation is:

> 'the sum of activity to ensure them the best possible physical, mental and social conditions so that they by their own efforts, regain as normal as possible a place in the community and lead an active productive life.'

In the 1960s observational studies on populations of working men rehabilitating and recovering from Myocardial Infarction (MI) largely focused on return to employment (Sharland 1964; Wincott 1966). Emerging experimental studies indicated the health benefits of exercise such as improved physical functioning, mood and self-confidence for patients following MI and those with angina (Gottheiner 1968; Kaufman and Anslow 1966). In the UK in 1970, Groden and colleagues (1971) captured the national picture of the limited cardiac rehabilitation available in Britain at that time, finding that only nine hospitals reported any form of exercise programme. Cardiologists responding to the survey were concerned that rehabilitation was being neglected, both in practice and teaching and called for greater education of medical undergraduates in the principles of rehabilitation and further trials of effective cardiac service models (Groden et al. 1971).

An overview of randomised controlled trials of cardiac rehabilitation for patients following MI conducted in the late 1980s highlighted the development of cardiac rehabilitation in many countries, particularly the US and in Europe (O'Connor et al. 1989). However, people older than 65–70 years and women had largely been excluded from these initial cardiac rehabilitation studies. For example, women constituted only 3% of the 4554 patients included in the 22 reviewed trials (O'Connor et al. 1989). In this early review, trials were classified as those providing 'exercise only' and 'exercise plus other interventions', highlighting distinctions between the exercise component of cardiac rehabilitation and other components such as lifestyle modifications, smoking cessation and interventions involving health professionals such as social workers, dieticians and psychologists. These multifactorial components and their psychosocial benefits remain recognisable in today's services.

Since the 1980s, research trials and services have continued to investigate the benefits of various components of cardiac rehabilitation including exercise, in more diverse groups of patients. These include patients following percutaneous coronary interventions (PCI), cardiac surgery, Coronary Artery Bypass Grafting (CABG), valve surgery, cardiac transplantation, and those diagnosed with heart failure, diabetes and peripheral vascular disease (Piepoli et al. 2010). These trials have informed evidence-based clinical guidelines that aim to raise standards of care for people with these conditions who could benefit from participation in cardiac rehabilitation. These guidelines, including the patient groups that should be invited to participate in cardiac rehabilitation, are discussed later in this chapter.

13.3 Cardiac Rehabilitation: The Evidence

In early 2018, the Danish Centre on Rehabilitation and Palliative Care in collaboration with the Cochrane Cardiac Rehabilitation Group at University of Exeter in England reviewed the evidence and gaps in rehabilitation and palliative care in the management of cardiovascular diseases (Joshi et al. 2018). Their broad 'review of reviews' focused specifically on systematic reviews and meta-analyses. They found an extensive body of evidence supporting the benefits of exercise-based rehabilitation in coronary heart disease (i.e. myocardial infarction and post-revascularisation) (Anderson et al. 2016; Uddin et al. 2016), heart failure(Taylor et al. 2014; Zhang et al. 2016; Chan et al. 2016) and intermittent claudication (Lane et al. 2014). Exercise capacity, health-related quality of life and risk of hospital admission were found to improve with exercise compared to no exercise control groups in these conditions.

Although earlier meta-analyses of the benefits of exercise-based cardiac rehabilitation among people with Coronary Heart Disease (CHD) indicated reductions in all-cause mortality (Jolliffe et al. 2001; Taylor et al. 2004), more recent analyses that included more mixed populations of people with CHD have found statistically significant reductions in CHD mortality, but not all-cause mortality (Anderson et al. 2016). This indicates that, in an era of optimal medical treatment, the opportunity for gains in overall mortality may be reduced. Furthermore, a recent meta-analysis re-examining the evidence of exercise-based cardiac rehabilitation using the same entry criterion as a previous Cochrane review (MI, CABG, PCI, angina pectoris and coronary artery disease) but limiting included studies from 2000 onwards (versus from 1975) to better reflect contemporary populations, found no effect on all-cause and CVD mortality and questioned whether the small reductions in hospital admissions found were clinically meaningful (Powell et al. 2018).

The impacts of exercise-based cardiac rehabilitation have been reviewed for stable angina (Long et al. 2018), heart valve surgery (Sibilitz et al. 2016), Transcatheter Aortic Valve Implantation (TAVI) (Ribeiro et al. 2017), pulmonary hypertension (Morris et al. 2017) and heart transplantation (Anderson et al. 2017). Overall, findings indicate evidence for improved exercise capacity among people with these conditions. However, there are fewer high-quality trials featuring adequate length of cardiac rehabilitation duration and study follow-up periods, compared with more prevalent cardiac conditions such as MI. One exception is the systematic review by Ribeiro and colleagues (2017) finding that in patients with Aortic Stenosis corrected by surgical aortic valve replacement or TAVI, an early post-surgical cardiac rehabilitation programme even of short duration (3 weeks) demonstrated improvements in exercise tolerance, functional independence, health-related quality of life and maximal exercise capacity. Among those with implantable cardioverter-defibrillators, a systematic review found exercise-based rehabilitation improved exercise capacity and reduce the likelihood of shocks (Pandey et al. 2017). Similarly, for those with atrial fibrillation (Risom et al. 2017) positive effects on physical exercise capacity resulted from cardiac rehabilitation, but the certainty of the magnitude of the effect could not be established due to the low number of patients and the low quality of some trials in the review. Joshi and colleagues (2018) reported finding no systematic reviews on the effectiveness of exercise interventions among conditions including infective endocarditis, cardiac arrest survivors, congenital heart disease, venous embolism and acute aortic syndrome. Further research is needed in these conditions and the current lack of evidence may not necessarily be indicative of a lack of efficacy.

13.3.1 Evidence Gaps for Frail Older People

Frailty is a comparatively recent concept when compared to the initial development and trials conducted in cardiac rehabilitation (Gielen and Simm 2017). Large trials that established the evidence for cardiac rehabilitation, particularly for MI, CABG and PCI, were conducted in an era when frailty assessment was not routinely undertaken, and study entry criteria did not always include older adults with multiple conditions. In the early 1990s, the benefits of exercise for those with heart failure was established, later than other cardiac disease (Coats et al. 1990). Older people with multiple morbidities represent a considerable proportion of those participating in cardiac rehabilitation in several countries (Giallauria et al. 2010; Foundation 2018; Menezes et al. 2014). Although heart failure research has tended to include older adults, and increasingly those with multimorbidity, studies specifically related to exercise and cardiac rehabilitation have not routinely characterised frailty (Taylor et al. 2018). Therefore, specific evidence for cardiac rehabilitation for frail older adults is limited for contemporary populations, despite them being a group that may potentially have the most to gain from this intervention (Singh et al. 2014).

A key consideration in the evidence for cardiac rehabilitation for frail older adults is the average age of adults included in trials, their comorbidities and specifically their frailty status, which to date, has largely been absent from the literature. Recognising some of the limitations of generalising previous trail data to older patients, Suaya and colleagues (2009) examined the one- to five-year mortality rates in a population of 601 099 patients, aged 65 years and over, who were hospitalised for coronary conditions or cardiac revascularisation procedures in the US. Mortality rates were 21–34% lower in those participating in cardiac rehabilitation and this study, based on routinely collected data, provides some evidence that mortality benefits may be associated with selected older populations (Suaya et al. 2009).

13.4 Recommendations on Who Should Attend Cardiac Rehabilitation

Many international guidelines have made recommendations about types of people and their cardiac conditions who should attend cardiac rehabilitation (Piepoli et al. 2016; Scottish Intercollegiate Guidelines Network (SIGN) 2017; British Association for Cardiovascular Prevention and Rehabilitation 2017; Yancy et al. 2017; Thomas et al. 2018; Smith et al. 2011; Woodruffe et al. 2015; Japanese Circulation Society (JCS) 2014; Herdy et al. 2014). Irrespective of age, sex and ethnic group many types of patients are suitable including those: with CHD (angina, acute coronary syndrome including MI); before and after revascularisation (percutaneous revascularisation or surgery); following a stepwise alteration in CHD condition; with other atherosclerotic disease (e.g. peripheral arterial disease); with stable heart failure and cardiomyopathy; with congenital heart disease and following implantable device interventions (British Association for Cardiovascular Prevention and

Rehabilitation 2017). These conditions are summarised in Box 1.

Box 1 Recommended patient groups for cardiac rehabilitation

- acute coronary syndrome (ACS)
- chronic coronary artery disease (CAD)
- coronary revascularization
- heart failure
- stable angina
- peripheral arterial disease and surgery of the great vessels
- post-cerebrovascular event
- post-implantation of pacemakers, cardiac defibrillators and resynchronisation devices
- post-heart valve repair/replacement
- post-heart transplantation and ventricular assist devices
- Adult Congenital Heart Disease (ACHD)

Source Summarised from British Association for Cardiovascular Prevention and Rehabilitation 2017 guidance and Secondary prevention in the clinical management of patients with cardiovascular diseases. Core components, standards and outcome measures for referral and delivery: A Policy Statement from the Cardiac Rehabilitation Section of the European Association for Cardiovascular Prevention & Rehabilitation 2014.

13.5 Contemporary Cardiac Rehabilitation Service Models

Cardiac rehabilitation services exist in just over half (55%) of countries throughout the world (Lima de Melo Ghisi et al. 2018), mostly in countries defined as high income by the World Bank (Turk-Adawi et al. 2014). Today's cardiac rehabilitation in many of these countries is a comprehensive, structured intervention that addresses the complex relationships of psychological, behavioural and medical factors confronting people with heart conditions (British Association for Cardiovascular Prevention and Rehabilitation 2017; Corra et al. 2005). Exercise training is a core component of cardiac rehabilitation and guidelines consistently recommend "comprehensive rehabilitation" programmes that include multifactorial components to optimise cardiovascular risk reduction, promote healthy behaviours and an active lifestyle, to reduce disability and improve health and wellbeing. Such programmes are designed to limit the physiological and psychological effects of cardiac illness, stabilise or reverse the atherosclerotic process, control and improve symptoms and reduce morbidity (Taylor 2015).

13.5.1 Core Components of Comprehensive Cardiac Rehabilitation

Core elements of comprehensive cardiac rehabilitation have been described in frequently cited guidance (British Association for Cardiovascular Prevention and Rehabilitation 2017; Piepoli et al. 2014; Balady et al. 2007). These are revised regularly but have some concepts in common. For example, the published standards on the core components of cardiac rehabilitation outlined by the British Association for Cardiovascular Prevention and Rehabilitation (BACPR) in 2017 are summarised in Table 13.1 (British Association for Cardiovascular Prevention and Rehabilitation 2017). Delivery of core components should be by a qualified and competent multidisciplinary team, led by a clinical coordinator. Health professionals leading each component (exercise, dietary and smoking cessation) should be appropriately qualified, skilled and competent. Recommended minimum standards for staffing a cardiac rehabilitation service have been described in some countries (Scottish Intercollegiate Guidelines Network (SIGN) 2017; British Association for Cardiovascular Prevention and Rehabilitation 2017). Although recommendations on programme duration remains an area of debate, it is generally accepted the comprehensive programmes should be a minimum of

Table 13.1 Core components for cardiac rehabilitation

Six core components	Description
Health behaviour change and education	Education sessions should include: addressing misconceptions about cardiac illness (and rehabilitation), lifestyle education, risk factor education such as blood pressure, lipids and glucose, occupational factors, sexual dysfunction, cardiopulmonary resuscitation and pharmaceutical and surgical interventions
Lifestyle risk factor management • Physical activity and exercise • Healthy eating and body composition • Tobacco cessation and relapse prevention	Baseline assessment should include: • physical fitness (to tailor exercise prescription/goals) • dietary habits, including adherence with a cardioprotective diet and alcohol use • measurement of weight, body mass index and waist circumference • medical advice to quit smoking should be reinforced and a quit plan discussed with repeat assessment of progress with cessation at every visit
Psychosocial health	All patients should undergo a valid assessment of: Psychological distress, Quality of life, Psychological stressors, Illness perceptions and self-efficacy for health behaviour change, Adequacy of social support, and have the opportunity to discuss to sexual health
Medical risk management	Assessment should include: Measurement of blood pressure, lipids, glucose, heart rate and rhythm; current medication use (dose and adherence). Best practice standards and guidelines should be followed Cardiovascular prevention and rehabilitation services also provide an opportunity to identify patients who may benefit from an implantable device
Long-term strategies	By the end of the programme patients will have been encouraged and empowered to develop self-management skills to pursue a healthy lifestyle
Audit and evaluation of services	To monitor and manage patient progress and service resources To evaluate programmes in terms of clinical and patient-reported outcomes To enable benchmarking against local, regional and national standards

Source Adapted from British Association for Cardiovascular Prevention and Rehabilitation (BACPR) (2017), pp. 11–18

8–12 weeks duration followed by opportunities for life-long behavioural change (British Association for Cardiovascular Prevention and Rehabilitation 2017; Piepoli et al. 2014). Included in this process of rehabilitation is cardiac education (including risk factor modification, lifestyle and medication advice, and how patients can deal with emergencies), support, psychological therapy and counselling. Cognitive behavioural methods are effective in supporting persons in adopting a healthy lifestyle and techniques such as motivational interviewing are recommended (Piepoli et al. 2016). A component on relaxation may be incorporated in the programme and discussions of areas such as anxiety, depression and stress management are considered integral to cardiac rehabilitation (Coats et al. 1995). Cardiac rehabilitation should be tailored to the individual's needs and the patient, carers and spouses should be involved in goal setting (British Association for Cardiovascular Prevention and Rehabilitation 2017).

13.5.2 Service Delivery Locations and Patients' Preferences

Cardiac rehabilitation varies internationally and is delivered in a variety of primary, secondary and tertiary care settings including hospitals (both as an inpatient and outpatient), community clinics and centres, and home environments and may involve telephone monitoring and internet-based services (Clark et al. 2015). In the UK, US and most European countries cardiac rehabilitation has traditionally been delivered to groups of patients in healthcare and community settings. Some European countries offering residential intensive programmes of 3–4 week duration whilst other outpatient programmes last 3–6 months (Menezes et al. 2014; Taylor 2015). By contrast, the UK offer less intensive programmes usually delivered in supervised outpatient groups in hospitals and community centres starting 2–4 weeks after PCI or MI and 4–6 weeks after cardiac surgery (Taylor 2015; Bethell et al. 2009).

Published reviews and meta-analyses on the effectiveness of cardiac rehabilitation service models have demonstrated that home and centre-based cardiac rehabilitation appeared equally effective in improving clinical and health-related quality of life outcomes in acute MI and revascularisation patients (Anderson et al. 2017). Trials of internet-based cardiac rehabilitation have shown promising findings for patients with angina (Devi et al. 2014) and self-management in CHD (Kerr et al. 2010). High quality web-based cardiac rehabilitation alternatives for those declining or dropping out of conventional rehabilitation have indicated positive effects for interventions of 6 month duration (Houchen-Wolloff et al. 2018). Technology-based interventions for patients participating in cardiac rehabilitation are explicitly recommended in some national guidelines (Scottish Intercollegiate Guidelines Network (SIGN) 2017).

Some studies have investigated older patients' preferences for cardiac rehabilitation service models (Buttery et al. 2014; Boyde et al. 2018; Tang et al. 2017). In a study of 106 heart failure inpatients (mean age 78 years, 62% male, 47% lived alone, 55% NYHA class III, 39% falls in past 6 months, mean Charlson Comorbidity Index 3.3 (SD 1.7)) admitted to elderly care, cardiology and general medicine wards in a large UK hospital, most patients (72%) wanted to attend cardiac rehabilitation, preferring group-based programmes at hospitals over community classes (Buttery et al. 2014). Mean grip strength, a valid indicator of frailty (Syddall et al. 2003), was low in this sample (women: mean 16.5 kg/m^2 (SD 6.3), men 25.3 kg/m^2 (SD 9.5). Patients emphasised that superior hospital facilities and equipment, such as defibrillators, and the availability of health professionals provided them with greater confidence to participate at hospitals. Those preferring hospital programmes were younger (mean 5.1 years, 95% CI –10.1 to –0.1, P = 0.043) than those preferring not to participate and neither disease severity nor co-morbidity was associated with preferences. However, in this hospital sample only 21% were referred to any cardiac rehabilitation service on discharge.

Findings from a study in Australia investigating patient preferences among inpatients also found that most strongly preferred a centre-based compared to a home-based program, starting within two (rather than six weeks) of hospital discharge and with exercise delivered in a group rather than an individual setting (Boyde et al. 2018). However, exercise via the internet using telehealth was strongly disliked, among this Australian study population and there was an overall preference against delivery by smart phone Apps. Studies in Europe have indicated that preferences for either a supervised centre-based setting, or a self-management home-based setting may be more equally preferred (Tang et al. 2017). Further studies exploring frail older patient's preferences for service models particularly around preferences for digital health options are required.

13.5.3 The Emerging Role of 'Prehab' for Older Adults

Elective cardiac patients are at risk of functional and psychological decline in the time preceding surgery and preoperative rehabilitation ('prehab') to reduce hospital length of stay for people undergoing CABG, valve repair/replacement (via sternotomy) and TAVI surgery using the Clinical Frailty Scale as an outcome have been investigated (Waite et al. 2017). In a prospective, single centre pilot study, patients were seen in pre-operative assessment clinics and were assessed using a battery of functional capacity measures including the 6-minute walk test (6MWT) (American Thoracic Society (ATS) 2002), the Duke Activity Status Index (DASI)

(Hlatky et al. 1989) and the Short Physical Performance (SPPB) (Guralnik et al. 1994). The home-based prehab exercise intervention was individually tailored by a specialist physiotherapist and included a 6-week programme of progressive balance and strength exercises performed 3 times per week and involved self-monitoring of exercise intensity using the Rating of Perceived Exercising scale (RPE) (Borg 1982). Pre- and post-intervention results showed improvements in frailty status and improved balance, strength and gait speed. Furthermore, using the Clinical Frailty Scale for baseline assessment and 6-week follow-up proved appropriate in this small study.

In a systematic review investigating the incidence of postoperative pulmonary complications among cardiac surgical patients, 17 trials including 2689 patients were identified (Snowdon et al. 2014). Pre-operative interventions varied and included exercise, respiratory training, breathing exercises, stress management, relaxation and varied by their model of delivery (e.g. pre-admission exercise/education booklet, video, group-sessions, sessions with a health professional and multidisciplinary training). Preoperative interventions were found to reduce post-operative complications, reduce the time to post-operative extubation, and reduced the length of stay for older patients (over the age of 63 years), but not younger patients, indicating that those with more complex health needs and co-morbidities may have the most benefit. The effects of inspiratory muscle training were particularly effective in reducing hospital length of stay (by mean 2.1 days) and the risk of post-operative complications (by 58%). To obtain these benefits, clinicians delivered inspiratory muscle training 6–7 times a week for two to four weeks (supervised once per week by a physiotherapist); starting at a resistance of 15–30% of maximal inspiratory pressure and increasing by 5% each session. Thirteen patients would need to be treated with inspiratory muscle training to prevent one postoperative pulmonary complication (Snowdon et al. 2014).

13.5.4 Cost-Effectiveness of Cardiac Rehabilitation Service Models

One final consideration in cardiac rehabilitation service models is determining their cost-effectiveness. Shields and colleagues conducted a systematic review to examine the cost-effectiveness of cardiac rehabilitation following the widespread introduction of statins and stenting (Shields et al. 2018). From the 19 studies included in this qualitative synthesis, they reported cardiac rehabilitation is cost effective in the modern era, especially when an exercise component is included, supporting two earlier economic reviews with similar findings (Papadakis et al. 2005; Wong et al. 2012). In the review, the authors noted that all the cost-effectiveness studies used life-years as an outcome, potentially underestimating the benefits of cardiac rehabilitation in reducing morbidity (Shields et al. 2018). One study, comparing a 3-month versus a 12-month programme found that overall the 3 month programme was more cost-effective (Papadakis et al. 2008). However, a sub-analysis in this two group cost-effectiveness analysis found the 3 month programme was more cost-effective for patients at high risk, those with previous CABG and for male patients, whilst the longer programme was more cost-effective for lower risk patients and for female patients, suggesting that improved cost-effectiveness may be gained by triaging patients to different cardiac rehabilitation service models (Papadakis et al. 2008).

In a Cochrane review comparing the effectiveness of home and centre-based service models, 6 of the 23 included trials reported costs (Anderson et al. 2017). Home-based and hospital- or centre-based cardiac rehabilitation were found to be of similar effectiveness in improving clinical and health-related quality of life (HRQoL) outcomes in patients after MI, revascularisation or with heart failure and there was a lack of evidence of differences in healthcare costs between these approaches. This finding supports recommendations about offering individual patient choice in service delivery models. Similarly, Shields and colleagues (Shields et al. 2018) reported that all studies comparing telehealth-based or assisted cardiac rehabilitation in their review found that these interventions were deemed cost-effective and noted that in practice, with increased patient numbers and economies of scale, cost may be further reduced.

13.5.5 Frailty Assessment in Cardiac Rehabilitation

Due to the epidemiology of certain age-related cardiac diagnoses, such as heart failure, that have a high average age of onset (Conrad et al. 2018) and procedures including implantable devices and interventions for degenerative valve disease that are largely undertaken among older adults (Ribeiro et al. 2017), frailty has been more frequently studied among these conditions. However, studies investigating relationships between certain cardiac conditions and frailty have been largely undertaken to characterise patients in hospital settings, for example the FRAIL-HF study, a prospective observational cohort study that was designed to evaluate clinical outcomes (mortality and readmission), functional evolution, quality of life, and use of social resources after hospital admission in Spain (Vidan et al. 2014). In terms of cardiac surgery, frailty assessment is often undertaken pre-operatively for risk stratification and prognostic purposes, and a recent review of 6 studies and 4756 patients undergoing cardiac surgery or TAVI found that frail older people have a higher risk of mortality, morbidity and functional decline regardless of the frailty assessment used (Sepehri et al. 2014). The European Association of Preventative Cardiology (EAPC) cardiac rehabilitation section has called for the use of standardised frailty assessment measures and suggested the Edmonton Frailty Scale (Rolfson et al. 2006) and the Clinical Frailty Scale from the CHSA study (Rockwood et al. 2005) as potentially suitable tools in cardiac rehabilitation services (Vigorito et al. 2017). Furthermore, the EAPC seek to evaluate the feasibility and timing of using frailty assessment tools in cardiac rehabilitation centres through a European registry study among people aged 75 years and over (Vigorito et al. 2017).

In a review of 61 studies relating to valve surgery and frailty (Tamuleviciute-Prasciene et al. 2018), a large range of frailty assessment tools were used including Fried phenotype frailty index and its modifications, multidimensional geriatric assessment, clinical frailty scale, 5 m walking test, serum albumin levels, and Katz Index of Independence of Activities of Daily Living. The AHA guidelines for the management of patients with valvular heart disease (Nishimura Rick et al. 2014, 2017) recommend the use of the Katz Index (independence in feeding, bathing, dressing, transferring, toileting, and urinary continence) and the 5 m gait speed test in assessment, with independence in ambulation classified as no walking aid or assist required, or being able to perform a 5 m walk test in less than 6 s (Nishimura Rick et al. 2014). As frailty status is dynamic over time, a single test may not be suitable to show the potential comprehensive effects of cardiac rehabilitation on those with frailty, and further studies are required to best understand the quickest, easiest and most sensitive frailty assessment tools for use in cardiac rehabilitation programmes (Tamuleviciute-Prasciene et al. 2018). Exercise-based cardiac rehabilitation for patients after aortic stenosis and interventional treatment have demonstrated improvements in Barthel index, Functional Independence Measure (FIM), 6MWT and anxiety and depression scales (Ribeiro et al. 2017). Using functional tools with established validity and reliability among frail older community dwelling adults (e.g. the Timed Up and Go, SPPB), may be useful in future studies of the effects of cardiac rehabilitation programmes. Measures that are often associated with falls risk and frailty, such as assessing self-reported number of falls in the previous 6 months, polypharmacy or measures of sarcopenia (e.g. chair-stand test) (Cruz-Jentoft et al. 2019) and nutritional status, which may improve with cardiac rehabilitation programmes should also be considered.

13.5.6 Exercise Prescription in Cardiac Rehabilitation for Frail Older Adults

Individual exercise prescription is a cornerstone of cardiac rehabilitation. People attending have increasingly varied cardiac conditions and often a broad range of co-morbidities. Exercises generally include a 'warm up', an aerobic exercise component (including exercising at the individual's target heart rate) and a 'cool down' period including muscle stretching exercises (Wenger 2008). The aerobic exercise component often consists of a series of exercises that suit being conducted in a circuit class; such as doing step ups and using exercise equipment such as an exercise bike.

A review on the consensus of international guidelines of exercise testing, prescription and monitoring in cardiac rehabilitation indicated there is large overlap between countries (Price et al. 2016). Cardiac rehabilitation societies in North and South America and Europe recommend electrocardiograph-monitored exercise stress tests and progress from moderate- to vigorous-intensity aerobic endurance exercise over the course of cardiac rehabilitation programmes and advise the inclusion of resistance training for maintaining independence and quality of life. However, those in the United Kingdom, Australia and New Zealand tend to specify lower-intensity exercise and less technical assessment of functional capacity (Price et al. 2016).

Specifically, for people with heart failure, recommendations have been made for the intensity of exercise prescribed. Exercises should ideally be performed at 60–80% of aerobic capacity and at 50% for more debilitated patients who may also require a longer warm-up period (Pina et al. 2003). Repeated lifting of significant weight should be avoided in people with heart failure due to the potential deleterious effects on ventricular function (Wenger 2008). Recommendations by the American Heart Association outline that exercise should be undertaken 3–5 times per week and should include supplementary walking and exercise on 'non-training days' (Pina et al. 2003). Evidence for exercise training for older frail people after cardiac surgeries and interventions for valvular disease indicates that training should be: individualised; measured by RPE, beginning at 40–60% of maximal VO_2; and include additional strength training by using the 1 repetition maximum method to prescribe intensity (Tamuleviciute-Prasciene et al. 2018).

Continuous aerobic exercise training (CAET) is a long-established mode of effective exercise training among those with CHD and a key feature of cardiac rehabilitation programmes. More recently, high-intensity interval training (HIIT), that includes alternating between high and low intense exercise during a training session, has emerged as an alternative or complementary exercise training method for CHD (Ribeiro et al. 2017). Among those with coronary artery disease, HIIT has been associated with greater gains in mean maximal VO_2 when compared with moderate intensity continuous training, whereas, moderate intensity continuous training has been associated with more marked declines in patients' mean resting heart rate and body weight than HITT (Liou et al. 2016). However, in relation to older adults, in a randomised controlled trail comparing HITT, resistance training, and combined exercise training between young (18–30 years) or older (65–80 years) adults, only HIIT improved aerobic capacity and skeletal muscle mitochondrial respiration, but leg strength did not change significantly with HIIT, and older adults may respond better to continuous training to improve maximal VO_2, compared to HIIT (Robinson et al. 2017). Finally, resistance training is a key intervention to improve sarcopenia (Cruz-Jentoft et al. 2019) and frailty (Skelton and Mavroeidi 2018), and ensuring sarcopenia detection and treatment is embedded in cardiac rehabilitation programmes for older adults requires a shift in focus from traditional CHD training regimes that tend to be more heavily weighted towards improving cardiorespiratory fitness parameters.

13.6 Referral, Invitation and Participation in Cardiac Rehabilitation

People with cardiovascular disease and frailty may encounter a wide variety of health professionals with varied knowledge and skills in primary and secondary care. These health professionals may be involved in recommending and inviting patients for cardiac rehabilitation. However, knowledge of cardiac rehabilitation guidelines differs between and within professional groups, as does the value that professionals place on guidelines and the influence they exert over their clinical practice (Remme et al. 2008). Some practitioners may initiate conversations with patients about the benefits of exercise and cardiac rehabilitation, but others may not identify this as a part of their role. This is a recognised issue, even within cardiac rehabilitation services, where nurses and physiotherapists view their roles differently (Thow et al. 2006). Cardiac rehabilitation nurses may be the first contact patients have with cardiac rehabilitation services in hospital (Thow et al. 2006), and these professionals play a key role in endorsing participation following referral (Jackson et al. 2005). Actively identifying all people potentially eligible for cardiac rehabilitation, and encouraging them to take part in cardiac rehabilitation prior to hospital discharge is a key clinical issue for those providing an effective cardiac rehabilitation service (Department of Health 2010).

13.6.1 Improving Referral to Cardiac Rehabilitation

Findings from England have shown that patients admitted to cardiology wards and those under the care of a specialist heart failure service, may be more likely to receive follow-up, such as cardiac rehabilitation (The NHS Information Centre 2010). Many healthcare systems rely on individual health professionals to refer patients to cardiac rehabilitation. These ad hoc systems result in missed opportunities to offer invitation. The first step to improve participation in cardiac rehabilitation for patients with frailty is the development of more systematic and system-wide referral processes.

Methods to improve cardiac rehabilitation referral using automatic electronic referral strategies, including electronic prompts, have proved effective in the US and Canada (Gravely-Witte et al. 2010; Grace et al. 2007; Mazzini et al. 2008). Combining electronic referral methods with evidence-based best-practice algorithms, standing orders and discharge checklists for patients may prove useful in both hospital and community settings to prompt referrals by clinicians. The availability of inpatient physical therapy has been found to be associated with higher rates of referral to cardiac rehabilitation (Mazzini et al. 2008). Involving professional groups, such as those that routinely discuss exercise and rehabilitation with patients in hospital and in the community, and investigating clinical decision tools and electronic referral methods may prove effective approaches for those with frailty. Using community-based risk stratification approaches to help identify those with frailty, such as the Electronic Frailty Index (eFI) (Clegg et al. 2016) may help identify older adults who may be undergoing annual reviews or other contacts with health professionals that could include opportunities for cardiac rehabilitation invitation.

13.6.2 Improving Invitation to Cardiac Rehabilitation

Sufficient information is required to enable a patient to make an informed choice and consent to a treatment (Charles et al. 1999). Communication of the benefits and the risks of an intervention are necessary. Service options need to be presented, so that decisions to opt for a certain intervention are shared between the patient and the health care provider (Charles et al. 1999). Providing a full explanation of cardiac rehabilitation, its components, benefits and the localities and service models available, is key for ensuring that patients are able to make an informed choice about participation.

Cardiac rehabilitation is effective in improving quality of life among patients with heart failure (Davies et al. 2010). This benefit should be emphasised at invitation. The risks associated with participation are minimal (Taylor 2015). Ensuring referral for older patients with cardiovascular disease and frailty and providing individually tailored invitation is essential for improving participation. Those inviting patients to participate must be knowledgeable of cardiac rehabilitation service components, the types of service models available and be able to confidently discuss the benefits of this intervention.

13.6.3 Improving Service Provision for Frail Older Adults

Globally, there is an overall lack of cardiac rehabilitation service availability and limited variety of service models for patients (Lima de Melo Ghisi et al. 2018). Furthermore, services may operate restricted provision to certain groups of patients with cardiovascular disease (Buttery et al. 2014); inconsistent with international guidance on the types of patients that should be offered and benefit from this intervention. Multidisciplinary cardiovascular clinics and services can take a leading role in providing some aspects of secondary prevention and care for patients with frailty. Strategies to facilitate closer working of these services to improve communication, referral and participation in supervised exercise that includes educational and psychological components for patients with frailty are required. Greater joint working, joint training opportunities and shared quality improvement initiatives between cardiology and geriatric services may help develop evidence-based services to better meet the needs of older people with cardiovascular disease and frailty.

13.7 Conclusion

This chapter has provided a summary of cardiac rehabilitation, from a brief historical context to the development of contemporary cardiac rehabilitation service delivery models. The core components of a cardiac rehabilitation programme were described and key research was highlighted, including large systematic reviews and cohort studies, which provide the evidence for clinical practice. These were discussed in the context of clinical guidelines and recommendations.

There is strong evidence of benefit of cardiac rehabilitation for patients with cardiovascular disease in terms of decreased morbidity. However, studies supporting this evidence were initially undertaken in selected younger populations and less frail people with cardiovascular disease compared to contemporary ageing populations. More recent studies are emerging in countries with older, frail populations that take into account the links between the research-based evidence for frailty interventions and cardiac rehabilitation components. Recognising the potential patient benefits on both frailty and cardiovascular disease trajectories, these studies have included measures of clinical frailty allowing new insights into this important and growing population. Patient identification, assessment, referral, invitation and choice in service provision are key areas for further investigation to allow more frail older people to potentially benefit from individually tailored cardiac rehabilitation programmes.

References

American Thoracic Society (ATS) (2002) Statement: guidelines for the six-minute walk test. Am J Respir Crit Care Med 166(1):111–117. https://doi.org/10.1164/ajrccm.166.1.at1102

Anderson L, Thompson DR, Oldridge N, Zwisler AD, Rees K, Martin N et al (2016) Exercise-based cardiac rehabilitation for coronary heart disease. The Cochrane Database Syst Rev (1):Cd001800. https://doi.org/10.1002/14651858.cd001800.pub3

Anderson L, Nguyen TT, Dall CH, Burgess L, Bridges C, Taylor RS (2017) Exercise-based cardiac rehabilitation in heart transplant recipients. Cochrane Database Syst Rev 4:Cd012264. https://doi.org/10.1002/14651858.cd012264.pub2

Anderson L, Sharp GA, Norton RJ, Dalal H, Dean SG, Jolly K et al (2017) Home-based versus centre-based cardiac rehabilitation. Cochrane Database Syst Rev 6:

Cd007130. https://doi.org/10.1002/14651858.cd007130.pub4

Balady GJ, Williams MA, Ades PA, Bittner V, Comoss P, Foody JM et al (2007) Core components of cardiac rehabilitation/secondary prevention programs: 2007 update. Circulation 115(20):2675–2682. https://doi.org/10.1161/CIRCULATIONAHA.106.180945

Bethell H, Lewin R, Dalal H (2009) Cardiac rehabilitation in the United Kingdom. Heart 95(4):271–275. https://doi.org/10.1136/hrt.2007.134338

Borg GA (1982) Psychophysical bases of perceived exertion. Med Sci Sports Exerc 14(5):377–381

Boyde M, Rankin J, Whitty JA, Peters R, Holliday J, Baker C et al (2018) Patient preferences for the delivery of cardiac rehabilitation. Patient Educ Couns 101(12):2162–2169. https://doi.org/10.1016/j.pec.2018.07.010

British Association for Cardiovascular Prevention and Rehabilitation (2017) The BACPR standards and core components for cardiovascular disease prevention and rehabilitation 2017 3rd edn, London UKBACPR

British Heart Foundation (2018) National audit of cardiac rehabilitation (NACR): quality and outcomes report 2018. https://www.bhf.org.uk/informationsupport/publications/statistics/national-audit-of-cardiac-rehabilitation-quality-and-outcomes-report-2018

Buttery AK, Carr-White G, Martin FC, Glaser K, Lowton K (2014a) Cardiac rehabilitation for heart failure: do older people want to attend and are they referred? Eur Geriatr Med 5(4):246–251. https://doi.org/10.1016/j.eurger.2014.04.011

Buttery AK, Carr-White G, Martin FC, Glaser K, Lowton K (2014b) Limited availability of cardiac rehabilitation for heart failure patients in the United Kingdom: findings from a national survey. Eur J Prev Cardiol 21(8):928–940. https://doi.org/10.1177/2047487313482286

Chan E, Giallauria F, Vigorito C, Smart NA (2016) Exercise training in heart failure patients with preserved ejection fraction: a systematic review and meta-analysis. Monaldi archives for chest disease = Archivio Monaldi per le malattie del torace 86(1–2):759. https://doi.org/10.4081/monaldi.2016.759

Charles C, Whelan T, Gafni A (1999) What do we mean by partnership in making decisions about treatment? Br Med J 319(7212):780–782

Clark RA, Conway A, Poulsen V, Keech W, Tirimacco R, Tideman P (2015) Alternative models of cardiac rehabilitation: a systematic review. Eur J Prev Cardiol 22(1):35–74. https://doi.org/10.1177/2047487313501093

Clegg A, Bates C, Young J, Ryan R, Nichols L, Ann Teale E et al (2016) Development and validation of an electronic frailty index using routine primary care electronic health record data. Age Ageing 45(3):353–360. https://doi.org/10.1093/ageing/afw039

Coats AJ, Adamopoulos S, Meyer TE, Conway J, Sleight P (1990) Effects of physical training in chronic heart failure. The Lancet 335(8681):63–66. https://doi.org/10.1016/0140-6736(90)90536-E

Coats A, McGee H, Stokes H, Thompson D (1995) British Association of Cardiac Rehabilitation: guidelines for cardiac rehabilitation. Blackwell Publishing, London

Conrad N, Judge A, Tran J, Mohseni H, Hedgecott D, Crespillo AP et al (2018) Temporal trends and patterns in heart failure incidence: a population-based study of 4 million individuals. The Lancet. 391(10120):572–580. https://doi.org/10.1016/S0140-6736(17)32520-5

Corra U, Giannuzzi P, Adamopoulos S, Bjornstad H, Bjarnason-Weherns B, Cohen-Solal A et al (2005) Executive summary of the position paper of the working group on cardiac rehabilitation and exercise physiology of the European Society of Cardiology (ESC): core components of cardiac rehabilitation in chronic heart failure. Eur J Cardiovasc Prev Rehabil 12(4):321–325

Cruz-Jentoft AJ, Bahat G, Bauer J, Boirie Y, Bruyère O, Cederholm T et al (2019) Sarcopenia: revised European consensus on definition and diagnosis. Age Ageing 48(1):16–31. https://doi.org/10.1093/ageing/afy169

Dalal HM, Doherty P, Taylor RS (2015) Cardiac rehabilitation. Br Med J 351. https://doi.org/10.1136/bmj.h5000

Davies EJ, Moxham T, Rees K, Singh S, Coats AJ, Ebrahim S et al (2010) Exercise based rehabilitation for heart failure. Cochrane Database Syst Rev 7:CD007131. https://doi.org/10.1002/14651858.cd003331.pub3

Department of Health (2010) Overview of commissioning cardiac rehabilitation services. Crown Copyright, Strategic Commissioning Development Unit, London

Devi R, Powell J, Singh S (2014) A web-based program improves physical activity outcomes in a primary care angina population: randomized controlled trial. J Med Internet Res 16(9):e186. https://doi.org/10.2196/jmir.3340

Dock W (1944) The evil sequelae of complete bed rest. JAMA: J Am Med Assoc 125(16):1083–1085. https://doi.org/10.1001/jama.1944.02850340009004

Giallauria F, Vigorito C, Tramarin R, Fattirolli F, Ambrosetti M, De Feo S et al (2010) Cardiac rehabilitation in very old patients: data from the Italian Survey on Cardiac Rehabilitation-2008 (ISYDE-2008)–official report of the Italian Association for Cardiovascular Prevention, Rehabilitation, and Epidemiology. J Gerontol Ser A, Biol Sci Med Sci 65(12):1353–1361. https://doi.org/10.1093/gerona/glq138

Gielen S, Simm A (2017) Frailty and cardiac rehabilitation: a long-neglected connection. Eur J Prev Cardiol 24(14):1488–1489. https://doi.org/10.1177/2047487317707842

Gottheiner V (1968) Long-range strenuous sports training for cardiac reconditioning and rehabilitation. Am J Cardiol 22(3):426–435. https://doi.org/10.1016/0002-9149(68)90126-4

Grace SL, Scholey P, Suskin N, Arthur HM, Brooks D, Jaglal S et al (2007) A prospective comparison of cardiac rehabilitation enrollment following automatic vs usual referral. J Rehabil Med 39:239–245

Gravely-Witte S, Leung YW, Nariani R, Tamim H, Oh P, Chan VM et al (2010) Effects of cardiac rehabilitation referral strategies on referral and enrollment rates. Nat Rev Cardiol 7(2):87–96

Groden BM, Semple T, Shaw GB (1971) Cardiac rehabilitation in Britain (1970). Br Heart J 33 (5):756–758. https://doi.org/10.1136/hrt.33.5.756

Guralnik JM, Simonsick EM, Ferrucci L, Glynn RJ, Berkman LF, Blazer DG et al (1994) A short physical performance battery assessing lower extremity function: association with self-reported disability and prediction of mortality and nursing home admission. J Gerontol 49(2):M85–M94

Heberden W (1802) Classics in cardiology: description of angina pectoris by William Heberden (London, T Payne, 1802). Heart Views 2006(7):118–119

Herdy AH, Lopez-Jimenez F, Terzic CP, Milani M, Stein R, Carvalho T et al (2014) South American guidelines for cardiovascular disease prevention and rehabilitation. Arq Bras Cardiol 103(2 Suppl 1):1–31

Hlatky MA, Boineau RE, Higginbotham MB, Lee KL, Mark DB, Califf RM et al (1989) A brief self-administered questionnaire to determine functional capacity (the Duke Activity Status Index). Am J Cardiol 64(10):651–654

Houchen-Wolloff L, Gardiner N, Devi R, Robertson N, Jolly K, Marshall T et al (2018) Web-based cardiac rehabilitation alternative for those declining or dropping out of conventional rehabilitation: results of the WREN feasibility randomised controlled trial. Open Heart 5(2):e000860-e. https://doi.org/10.1136/openhrt-2018-000860

Jackson L, Leclerc J, Erskine Y, Linden W (2005) Getting the most out of cardiac rehabilitation: a review of referral and adherence predictors. Heart 91(1):10–14. https://doi.org/10.1136/hrt.2004.045559

Japanese Circulation Society (JCS) Joint Working Group (2014) Guidelines for rehabilitation in patients with cardiovascular disease (JCS 2012). Circ J 78(8):2022–2093. https://doi.org/10.1253/circj.cj-66-0094

Jolliffe J, Rees K, Taylor R, Thompson D, Oldridge N, Ebrahim S (2001) Exercise-based rehabilitation for coronary heart disease. Cochrane Database Syst Rev 1:CD001800. https://doi.org/10.1002/14651858.cd001800

Joshi V, Tang L, Long L, Zwisler AD, Taylor R (2018) Report on rehabilitation and palliative care in the management of cardiovascular diseases: the evidence and the gaps. REHPA, Danish Centre on Rehabilitation and Palliative Care

Kaufman JM, Anslow RD (1966) Treatment of refractory angina pectoris with nitroglycerin and graded exercise. JAMA: J Am Med Assoc 196(2):151–155

Kerr C, Murray E, Noble L, Morris R, Bottomley C, Stevenson F et al (2010) The potential of web-based interventions for heart disease self-management: a mixed methods investigation. J Med Internet Res 2:12 (4). https://www.jmir.org/2010/4/e56/

Lane R, Ellis B, Watson L, Leng GC (2014) Exercise for intermittent claudication. Cochrane Database Syst Rev (7):Cd000990. https://doi.org/10.1002/14651858.cd000990.pub3

Levine SA, Lown B (1952) “armchair” treatment of acute coronary thrombosis. J Am Med Assoc 148(16): 1365–1369. https://doi.org/10.1001/jama.1952.02930160001001

Lima de Melo Ghisi G, Pesah E, Turk-Adawi K, Supervia M, Lopez Jimenez F, Grace S (2018) Cardiac rehabilitation models around the globe. J Clin Med 7(9):260

Liou K, Ho S, Fildes J, Ooi S-Y (2016) High intensity interval versus moderate intensity continuous training in patients with coronary artery disease: a meta-analysis of physiological and clinical parameters. Heart, Lung Circ 25(2):166–174. https://doi.org/10.1016/j.hlc.2015.06.828

Long L, Anderson L, Dewhirst AM, He J, Bridges C, Gandhi M et al (2018) Exercise-based cardiac rehabilitation for adults with stable angina. Cochrane Database Syst Rev 2:Cd012786. https://doi.org/10.1002/14651858.cd012786.pub2

Mazzini MJ, Stevens GR, Whalen D, Ozonoff A, Balady GJ (2008) Effect of an American Heart Association get with the guidelines program-based clinical pathway on referral and enrollment into cardiac rehabilitation after acute myocardial infarction. Am J Cardiol 101(8):1084–1087

Menezes AR, Lavie CJ, Milani RV, Forman DE, King M, Williams MA (2014) Cardiac rehabilitation in the United States. Prog Cardiovasc Dis 56(5):522–529. https://doi.org/10.1016/j.pcad.2013.09.018

Morris NR, Kermeen FD, Holland AE (2017) Exercise-based rehabilitation programmes for pulmonary hypertension. Cochrane Database Syst Rev 1:Cd011285. https://doi.org/10.1002/14651858.cd011285.pub2

Nishimura Rick A, Otto Catherine M, Bonow Robert O, Carabello Blase A, Erwin John P, Guyton Robert A et al (2014) 2014 AHA/ACC guideline for the management of patients with valvular heart disease. Circulation 129(23):e521–e643. https://doi.org/10.1161/CIR.0000000000000031

Nishimura Rick A, Otto Catherine M, Bonow Robert O, Carabello Blase A, Erwin John P, Fleisher Lee A et al (2017) 2017 AHA/ACC focused update of the 2014 AHA/ACC guideline for the management of patients with valvular heart disease: a report of the American College of Cardiology/American Heart Association task force on clinical practice guidelines. Circulation 135(25):e1159–e1195. https://doi.org/10.1161/CIR.0000000000000503

O’Connor G, Buring J, Yusuf S, Goldhaber S, Olmstead E, Paffenbarger R Jr et al (1989) An overview of randomized trials of rehabilitation with exercise after myocardial infarction. Circulation 80(2):234–244

Pandey A, Parashar A, Moore C, Ngo C, Salahuddin U, Bhargava M et al (2017) Safety and efficacy of exercise training in patients with an implantable cardioverter-defibrillator: a meta-analysis. JACC: Clin Electrophysiol 3(2):117–126. https://doi.org/10.1016/j.jacep.2016.06.008

Papadakis S, Oldridge NB, Coyle D, Mayhew A, Reid RD, Beaton L et al (2005) Economic evaluation of cardiac rehabilitation: a systematic review. Eur J Cardiovasc Prev Rehabil 12(6):513–520

Papadakis S, Reid RD, Coyle D, Beaton L, Angus D, Oldridge N (2008) Cost-effectiveness of cardiac rehabilitation program delivery models in patients at varying cardiac risk, reason for referral, and sex. Eur J Cardiovasc Prev Rehabil 15(3):347–353. https://doi.org/10.1097/HJR.0b013e3282f5ffab

Piepoli MF, Corra U, Benzer W, Bjarnason-Wehrens B, Dendale P, Gaita D et al (2010) Secondary prevention through cardiac rehabilitation: from knowledge to implementation. A position paper from the cardiac rehabilitation section of the European Association of Cardiovascular Prevention and Rehabilitation. Eur J Cardiovasc Prev Rehabil 17(1):1–17. https://doi.org/10.1097/hjr.0b013e3283313592

Piepoli MF, Corra U, Adamopoulos S, Benzer W, Bjarnason-Wehrens B, Cupples M et al (2014) Secondary prevention in the clinical management of patients with cardiovascular diseases. Core components, standards and outcome measures for referral and delivery: a policy statement from the cardiac rehabilitation section of the European Association for Cardiovascular Prevention & Rehabilitation. Endorsed by the Committee for Practice Guidelines of the European Society of Cardiology. Eur J Prev Cardiol 21(6):664–681. https://doi.org/10.1177/2047487312449597

Piepoli MF, Hoes AW, Agewall S, Albus C, Brotons C, Catapano AL et al (2016) 2016 European guidelines on cardiovascular disease prevention in clinical practice the sixth joint task force of the European Society of Cardiology and other societies on cardiovascular disease prevention in clinical practice (constituted by representatives of 10 societies and by invited experts) developed with the special contribution of the European Association for Cardiovascular Prevention; Rehabilitation (EACPR). Eur Heart J 37(29):2315–2381. https://doi.org/10.1093/eurheartj/ehw106

Pina IL, Apstein CS, Balady GJ, Belardinelli R, Chaitman BR, Duscha BD et al (2003) Exercise and heart failure: a statement from the American Heart Association committee on exercise, rehabilitation, and prevention. Circulation 107(8):1210–1225. https://doi.org/10.1161/01.cir.0000055013.92097.40

Powell R, McGregor G, Ennis S, Kimani PK, Underwood M (2018) Is exercise-based cardiac rehabilitation effective? a systematic review and meta-analysis to re-examine the evidence. BMJ Open 8(3):e019656. https://doi.org/10.1136/bmjopen-2017-019656

Price KJ, Gordon BA, Bird SR, Benson AC (2016) A review of guidelines for cardiac rehabilitation exercise programmes: is there an international consensus? Eur J Prev Cardiol 23(16):1715–1733. https://doi.org/10.1177/2047487316657669

Remme WJ, McMurray JJV, Hobbs FDR, Cohen-Solal A, Lopez-Sendon J, Boccanelli A et al (2008) Awareness and perception of heart failure among European cardiologists, internists, geriatricians, and primary care physicians. Eur Heart J 29(14):1739–1752. https://doi.org/10.1093/eurheartj/ehn196

Ribeiro GS, Melo RD, Deresz LF, Dal Lago P, Pontes MR, Karsten M (2017) Cardiac rehabilitation programme after transcatheter aortic valve implantation versus surgical aortic valve replacement: Systematic review and meta-analysis. Eur J Prev Cardiol 24(7):688–697. https://doi.org/10.1177/2047487316686442

Ribeiro PAB, Boidin M, Juneau M, Nigam A, Gayda M (2017) High-intensity interval training in patients with coronary heart disease: prescription models and perspectives. Ann Phys Rehabil Med 60(1):50–57. https://doi.org/10.1016/j.rehab.2016.04.004

Risom SS, Zwisler AD, Johansen PP, Sibilitz KL, Lindschou J, Gluud C et al (2017) Exercise-based cardiac rehabilitation for adults with atrial fibrillation. Cochrane Database Syst Rev 2:Cd011197. https://doi.org/10.1002/14651858.cd011197.pub2

Robinson MM, Dasari S, Konopka AR, Johnson ML, Manjunatha S, Esponda RR et al (2017) Enhanced protein translation underlies improved metabolic and physical adaptations to different exercise training modes in young and old humans. Cell Metab 25(3):581–592. https://doi.org/10.1016/j.cmet.2017.02.009

Rockwood K, Song X, MacKnight C, Bergman H, Hogan DB, McDowell I et al (2005) A global clinical measure of fitness and frailty in elderly people. CMAJ: Can Med Assoc J = J de l'Association medicale canadienne 173(5):489–495. https://doi.org/10.1503/cmaj.050051

Rolfson DB, Majumdar SR, Tsuyuki RT, Tahir A, Rockwood K (2006) Validity and reliability of the Edmonton Frail Scale. Age Ageing 35(5):526–529. https://doi.org/10.1093/ageing/afl041

Scottish Intercollegiate Guidelines Network (SIGN) Cardiac rehabilitation. Edinburgh: SIGN; 2017. (SIGN publication no. 150). http://www.sign.ac.uk

Sepehri A, Beggs T, Hassan A, Rigatto C, Shaw-Daigle C, Tangri N et al (2014) The impact of frailty on outcomes after cardiac surgery: a systematic review. J Thorac Cardiovasc Surg 148(6):3110–3117. https://doi.org/10.1016/j.jtcvs.2014.07.087

Sharland D (1964) Ability of men to return to work after myocardial infarction. BMJ 2:718–720

Shields GE, Wells A, Doherty P, Heagerty A, Buck D, Davies LM (2018) Cost-effectiveness of cardiac rehabilitation: a systematic review. Heart 104(17):1403–1410. https://doi.org/10.1136/heartjnl-2017-312809

Sibilitz KL, Berg SK, Tang LH, Risom SS, Gluud C, Lindschou J et al (2016) Exercise-based cardiac rehabilitation for adults after heart valve surgery. Cochrane Database Syst Rev 3:Cd010876. https://doi.org/10.1002/14651858.cd010876.pub2

Singh M, Stewart R, White H (2014) Importance of frailty in patients with cardiovascular disease. Eur Heart J 35(26):1726–1731. https://doi.org/10.1093/eurheartj/ehu197

Skelton DA, Mavroeidi A (2018) Which strength and balance activities are safe and efficacious for individuals with specific challenges (osteoporosis, vertebral fractures, frailty, dementia)?: a narrative review. J Frailty, Sarcopenia Falls 3(2):85–104. https://doi.org/10.22540/jfsf-03-085

Smith SC, Benjamin EJ, Bonow RO, Braun LT, Creager MA, Franklin BA et al (2011) AHA/ACCF secondary prevention and risk reduction therapy for patients with coronary and other atherosclerotic vascular disease: 2011 update. A guideline from the American Heart Association and American College of Cardiology Foundation. Endorsed by the World Heart Federation and the Preventive Cardiovascular Nurses Association. J Am Coll Cardiol 58(23):2432–2446. https://doi.org/10.1016/j.jacc.2011.10.824

Snowdon D, Haines TP, Skinner EH (2014) Preoperative intervention reduces postoperative pulmonary complications but not length of stay in cardiac surgical patients: a systematic review. J Physiother 60(2):66–77. https://doi.org/10.1016/j.jphys.2014.04.002

Stewart S, MacIntyre K, Hole DJ, Capewell S, McMurray JJV (2001) More "malignant" than cancer? Five-year survival following a first admission for heart failure. Eur J Heart Fail 3(3):315–322. https://doi.org/10.1016/s1388-9842(00)00141-0

Suaya JA, Stason WB, Ades PA, Normand S-LT, Shepard DS (2009) Cardiac rehabilitation and survival in older coronary patients. J Am Coll Cardiol 54 (1):25–33. https://doi.org/10.1016/j.jacc.2009.01.078

Syddall H, Cooper C, Martin F, Briggs R, Aihie SA (2003) Is grip strength a useful single marker of frailty? Age Ageing 32(6):650–656. https://doi.org/10.1093/ageing/afg111

Tamuleviciute-Prasciene E, Drulyte K, Jurenaite G, Kubilius R, Bjarnason-Wehrens B (2018) Frailty and Exercise training: how to provide best care after cardiac surgery or intervention for elder patients with valvular heart disease. Biomed Res Int 2018:9849475. https://doi.org/10.1155/2018/9849475

Tang LH, Kikkenborg Berg S, Christensen J, Lawaetz J, Doherty P, Taylor RS et al (2017) Patients' preference for exercise setting and its influence on the health benefits gained from exercise-based cardiac rehabilitation. Int J Cardiol 232:33–39. https://doi.org/10.1016/j.ijcard.2017.01.126

Taylor RS, Brown A, Ebrahim S, Jolliffe J, Noorani H, Rees K et al (2004) Exercise-based rehabilitation for patients with coronary heart disease: systematic review and meta-analysis of randomized controlled trials. Am J Med 116(10):682–692. https://doi.org/10.1016/j.amjmed.2004.01.009

Taylor RS, Sagar VA, Davies EJ, Briscoe S, Coats AJS, Dalal H et al (2014) Exercise-based rehabilitation for heart failure. Cochrane Database Syst Rev (4). https://doi.org/10.1002/14651858.cd003331.pub4

Taylor RS, Walker S, Smart NA, Piepoli MF, Warren FC, Ciani O et al (2018) Impact of exercise-based cardiac rehabilitation in patients with heart failure (ExTraMATCH II) on mortality and hospitalisation: an individual patient data meta-analysis of randomised trials. Eur J Heart Fail. https://doi.org/10.1002/ejhf.1311

The NHS Information Centre (2010) National Heart Failure Audit 2010. Leeds: The NHS Information Centre for Health and Social Care

Thomas RJ, Balady G, Banka G, Beckie TM, Chiu J, Gokak S et al (2018) 2018 ACC/AHA Clinical performance and quality measures for cardiac rehabilitation. A report of the American College of Cardiology/American Heart Association Task Force on Performance Measures. J Am Coll Cardiol 71(16):1814–1837. https://doi.org/10.1016/j.jacc.2018.01.004

Thow MK, Rafferty D, McKay J (2006) National survey of the level of nursing involvement and the perceived skills and attributes required in the delivery of cardiac rehabilitation. Br J Cardiol 13:53–55

Turk-Adawi K, Sarrafzadegan N, Grace SL (2014) Global availability of cardiac rehabilitation. Nat Rev Cardiol 11(10):586–596. https://doi.org/10.1038/nrcardio.2014.98

Uddin J, Zwisler AD, Lewinter C, Moniruzzaman M, Lund K, Tang LH et al (2016) Predictors of exercise capacity following exercise-based rehabilitation in patients with coronary heart disease and heart failure: a meta-regression analysis. Eur J Prev Cardiol 23(7):683–693. https://doi.org/10.1177/2047487315604311

Vidan MT, Sanchez E, Fernandez-Aviles F, Serra-Rexach JA, Ortiz J, Bueno H (2014) FRAIL-HF, a study to evaluate the clinical complexity of heart failure in nondependent older patients: rationale, methods and baseline characteristics. Clin Cardiol 37(12):725–732. https://doi.org/10.1002/clc.22345

Vigorito C, Abreu A, Ambrosetti M, Belardinelli R, Corrà U, Cupples M et al (2017) Frailty and cardiac rehabilitation: a call to action from the EAPC cardiac rehabilitation section. Eur J Prev Cardiol 24(6):577–590. https://doi.org/10.1177/2047487316682579

Waite I, Deshpande R, Baghai M, Massey T, Wendler O, Greenwood S (2017) Home-based preoperative rehabilitation (prehab) to improve physical function and reduce hospital length of stay for frail patients undergoing coronary artery bypass graft and valve surgery. J Cardiothorac Surg 12(1):91. https://doi.org/10.1186/s13019-017-0655-8

Wenger NK (2008) Current status of cardiac rehabilitation. J Am Coll Cardiol 51(17):1619–1631. https://doi.org/10.1016/j.jacc.2008.01.030

West R (2004) Cardiac rehabilitation of older patients. Rev Clin Gerontol 13(03):241–255

Wincott EA (1966) Return to work after myocardial infarction. Br Med J 2:1302–1304. https://doi.org/10.1136/bmj.2.5525.1302

Wong WP, Feng J, Pwee KH, Lim J (2012) A systematic review of economic evaluations of cardiac rehabilitation. BMC Health Serv Res 12:243. https://doi.org/10.1186/1472-6963-12-243

Woodruffe S, Neubeck L, Clark RA, Gray K, Ferry C, Finan J et al (2015) Australian Cardiovascular Health and Rehabilitation Association (ACRA) core components of cardiovascular disease secondary prevention and cardiac rehabilitation 2014. Heart, Lung Circ 24(5):430–441. https://doi.org/10.1016/j.hlc.2014.12.008

World Health Organisation (1964) Rehabilitation of patients with cardiovascular diseases: report of a WHO Expert Committee. Geneva: Technical Report Series, No. 270

Yancy CW, Jessup M, Bozkurt B, Butler J, Casey DE Jr, Colvin MM et al (2017) 2017 ACC/AHA/HFSA focused update of the 2013 ACCF/AHA guideline for the management of heart failure: a report of the American College of Cardiology/American Heart Association Task Force on Clinical Practice Guidelines and the Heart Failure Society of America. Circulation 136(6):e137–e161. https://doi.org/10.1161/cir.0000000000000509

Zhang Y, Xu L, Yao Y, Guo X, Sun Y, Zhang J et al (2016) Effect of short-term exercise intervention on cardiovascular functions and quality of life of chronic heart failure patients: a meta-analysis. J Exerc Sci Fit 14(2):67–75. https://doi.org/10.1016/j.jesf.2016.08.001

Future Perspectives on the Role of Frailty in Cardiovascular Diseases

14

Timo E. Strandberg and Tuomo Nieminen

Abstract

Frailty is a clinical concept which is gaining increased momentum not only in geriatrics, but in all specialties treating adult patients. In these Future Perspectives, the following roles of frailty in the field of cardiovascular diseases (CVD) will be discussed as a narrative review: (1) Frailty as an adjunct to assess CVD patients in addition to traditional risk scores; (2) bidirectional relationship between frailty and CVD; (3) widening the scope of endpoints in CVD trials—inclusion of frailty; (4) finally, the relationship between geriatrics and cardiology will be shortly discussed.

Keywords

Frailty · Prognosis · Cardiovascular disease · Geriatrics · Perspective

T. E. Strandberg (✉)
University of Helsinki and Helsinki University Hospital, Haartmaninkatu 4, PO Box 340, FI-00029 Helsinki, Finland
e-mail: timo.strandberg@oulu.fi

Center for Life Course Health Research, University of Oulu, Oulu, Finland

T. Nieminen
Department of Internal Medicine of University of Helsinki, Helsinki University Hospital and Päijät Häme Central Hospital, Helsinki, Lahti, Finland

14.1 Use of Frailty as an Adjunct to Assess CVD Patients in Addition to Traditional Risk Scores Will Increase

Various ways and scores have been developed to help in the assessment of severity and prognosis of CVD patients. Besides "eyeball test", common examples are the New York Heart Association (NYHA) classification based on heart failure symptoms, and the CHA_2DS_2-VASc score using patient history to assess risk of stroke due to atrial fibrillation. There is clear evidence that the presence of frailty incrementally increases complication risk, including mortality, and assessment of frailty can thus give information over the disease specific risk scores (Afilalo et al. 2014).

However, inclusion of frailty assessments have been hampered by lack of knowledge of frailty and fears that it would burden busy clinicians by one more task. However, clinical systems and nurses already routinely collect essential information to be harnessed for the assessment of frailty status. In a British study, the Hospital Frailty Risk Score (HFRS) was established using various diagnoses associated with frailty (Gilbert et al. 2018), whereafter it was tested in a large validation cohort and shown to predict mortality, long hospital stay, and 30-day readmission. HFRS might offer a low-cost way for health systems to screen, for example, CVD patients with frailty for closer scrutiny with more time-consuming comprehensive geriatric

N. Veronese (ed.), *Frailty and Cardiovascular Diseases*, Advances in Experimental Medicine and Biology 1216, https://doi.org/10.1007/978-3-030-33330-0_14

assessment (CGA). Frailty screening may well be integral in future health care systems, although best ways for the implementation (e.g. frailty definition) still require more research.

14.2 Bidirectional Relationship Between Frailty and CVD Will Be Better Acknowledged

According to a meta-analysis, frailty and even pre-frailty are independent risk factors for CVD (Veronese et al. 2017). Evidently, development of frailty deteriorates the condition of a patient with existing CVD. Frailty is often associated with undernutrition, weight loss, and also with decreased physical activity, which is a CVD risk factor. Increase of physical activity is a treatment which would benefit both frailty and CVD. Improving nutrition in the case of weight loss is a complex question, because fortified diet should provide calories and protein but not worsen vascular status. Mediterranean diet has actually been associated with lower risk of incident frailty (Kojima et al. 2018), and thus olive oil and polyunsaturated fats should be preferred over butter and cream. For a patient with sarcopenic obesity (fat-frail), on the other hand, reducing overweight, which is beneficial for the heart, may be detrimental to muscles and thus promote sarcopenia, and should be performed carefully and with proper nutritional knowledge.

It is a scientifically intriguing question whether vascular factors promote frailty. In this discussion, frailty as a phenotype (Fried et al. 2001) is more interesting than frailty defined as an accumulation of defects (Searle et al. 2008), because CVD is already included in the latter and the relationships are obvious. Downstream it is easy to understand that established coronary heart disease or heart failure may accelerate sarcopenia and frailty by reducing physical activity. Pathophysiological factors such as inflammation related to CVD may also be involved. Cardiac cachexia is a special case related to terminal heart failure.

Cross-sectionally, frailty is associated with vascular risk factors (Ramsay et al. 2015), but less studied is the area whether vascular function is a long-term risk factor of frailty. Subclinical atherosclerosis has been associated with development of frailty (Chaves et al. 2004), and even longer-term associations with CVD risk factors have been described. In the Helsinki Businessmen Study, CVD risk factors such as overweight and physical inactivity in healthy midlife (at an average age of 47 years) predicted the development of frailty phenotype in old age, decades later (Strandberg et al. 2012; Savela et al. 2013). In a very large British study including the Clinical Practice Research Datalink (CPRD) and UK Biobank (UKB) data, CVD risk score was based on smoking status, LDL cholesterol, blood pressure, body mass index, fasting glucose, and physical activity. The score stratified 60–69 year old people to low, moderate or high CVD risk. During up to 10 years of follow-up, individuals with low CVD risk had substantially lower incidence of frailty and other geriatric conditions (Atkins JL et al. 2018).

Bidirectional relationships suggest that CVD and frailty have common antecedents, and this should be realized for better prevention of frailty. Proposed mechanisms for the CVD-frailty link usually include inflammation, oxidative stress, telomere shortening etc. (Stewart 2019). Adequate blood circulation is essential for all tissues, including muscle and brain, and factors deteriorating circulation via endothelial dysfunction and atherosclerotic lesions are excellent candidates to promote both physical and cognitive frailty. Large and especially small blood vessels are involved in the process (Strandberg et al. 2013).

14.3 Frailty Will Be Included as an Important Endpoint and Pre-specified Subgroup in All CVD Trials

Because risk factors predict frailty, elimination of risk factors is prone to prevent frailty, but controlled treatment trials are needed to verify the rationale. However, gathering geriatric endpoints like dementia or frailty can be difficult in CVD prevention trials, because study designs prefer relatively short follow-ups, and, for ethical reasons, the studies are still often terminated early due to rapid reduction of myocardial infarctions and stroke. Surrogate markers like change of biomarkers related to nutritional status or biological ageing (Stewart 2019), deterioration of physical function with sensitive tests, or progress of sarcopenia in imaging studies might be considered acceptable endpoints.

An important aspect is to pre-specify frailty as a subgroup in all CVD trials in order to find out whether main trial results also apply to frail participants (who should be included in trial populations!). Indeed, this was done in two hypertension trials, Hypertension in the Very Elderly Trial (HYVET, Warwick et al. 2015) and Systolic Blood Pressure Intervention Trial (SPRINT, Williamson et al. 2016), which showed that also at least moderately frail patients benefited from antihypertensive treatment. On the other hand, frail patients (defined by gait speed in the lowest tertile) seemed to have no mortality benefit from an implantable defibrillator in the Sudden Cardiac Death in Heart Failure Trial (SCD-HeFT, Fishbein et al. 2014), and in the Surgical Treatment for Ischemic Heart Failure (STICH) trial, shorter walk distance (<300 m) was not associated with long-term benefit from coronary artery bypass surgery (Stewart et al. 2014).

14.4 Cardiogeriatrics or Geriatric Cardiology

As successful primary prevention reduces premature CVD mortality, cardiology is increasingly a discipline involving older patients, of whom over 50% may be frail and need multidisciplinary care. Usually the latter part marks the emphasis in the names of medical specialities (e.g. psychogeriatrics versus geropsychiatry) . Because cardiology includes invasive skills not handled by geriatricians, geriatric cardiologist may be the appropriate term for future specialists who are able to embrace the multidimensional vulnerabilities and needs—medical, functional, cognitive, and social—of their older patients with CVD (Dodson et al. 2016; Gorodeski et al. 2018).

14.5 Conclusions

Cardiovascular diseases and frailty have an intimate relationship with common antecedents, and in the future, frailty will play an ever increasing role in the assessment and treatment of older cardiovascular patients. Conversely, finding better ways to prevent and treat frailty will benefit also patients with cardiovascular diseases. More research with novel trial settings are needed in this important field.

References

Afilalo J, Alexander KP, Mack MJ et al (2014) Frailty assessment in the cardiovascular care of older adults. J Am Coll Cardiol 63:747–762

Atkins JL, Delgado J, Pilling LC, Bowman K, Masoli JAH, Kuchel GA et al (2018) Impact of low cardiovascular risk profiles on geriatric outcomes: evidence from 421,000 participants in two cohorts. J Gerontol A Biol Sci Med Sci. https://doi.org/10.1093/gerona/gly083

Chaves PH, Kuller LH, O'Leary DH, Manolio TA, Newman AB (2004) Cardiovascular health study. Subclinical cardiovascular disease in older adults: insights from the cardiovascular health study. Am J Geriatr Cardiol 13:137–151

Dodson JA, Matlock DD, Forman DE (2016) Geriatric cardiology: an emerging discipline. Can J Cardiol 32:1056–1064

Fishbein DP, Hellkamp AS, Mark DB, Walsh MN, Poole JE, Anderson J et al (2014) SCD-HeFT investigators. Use of the 6-min walk distance to identify variations in treatment benefits from implantable cardioverter-defibrillator and amiodarone: results from the SCD-HeFT (Sudden Cardiac Death in Heart Failure Trial). J Am Coll Cardiol 63:2560–2568

Fried LP, Tangen CM, Walston J et al (2001) Cardiovascular health study collaborative research group. Frailty in older adults: evidence for a phenotype. J Gerontol A Biol Sci Med Sci 56:146–156

Gilbert T, Neuburger J, Kraindler J et al (2018) Development and validation of a hospital frailty risk score focusing on older people in acute care settings using electronic hospital records: an observational study. Lancet 391:1775–1782

Gorodeski EZ, Goyal P, Hummel SL et al (2018) Domain management approach to heart failure in the geriatric patient. Present and future. J Am Coll Cardiol. 71:1921–1936

Kojima G, Avgerinou C, Iliffe S, Walters K (2018) Adherence to mediterranean diet reduces incident frailty risk: systematic review and meta-analysis. J Am Geriatr Soc 66:783–788

Ramsay SE, Arianayagam DS, Whincup PH, Lennon LT, Cryer J, Papacosta AO et al (2015) Cardiovascular risk profile and frailty in a population-based study of older British men. Heart 101:616–622

Savela SL, Koistinen P, Stenholm S, Tilvis RS, Strandberg AY, Pitkälä KH et al (2013) Leisure-time physical activity in midlife is related to old age frailty. J Gerontol A Biol Sci Med Sci 68:1433–1438

Searle SD, Mitnitski A, Gahbauer EA, Gill TM, Rockwood K (2008) A standard procedure for creating a frailty index. BMC Geriatr 8:24. https://doi.org/10.1186/1471-2318-8-24

Stewart R (2019) Cardiovascular disease and frailty: what are the mechanistic links? Clin Chem 65:ePub

Stewart RA, Szalewska D, She L, Lee KL, Drazner MH, Lubiszewska B et al (2014) Exercise capacity and mortality in patients with ischemic left ventricular dysfunction randomized to coronary artery bypass graft surgery or medical therapy: an analysis from the STICH trial (Surgical Treatment for Ischemic Heart Failure). J Am Coll Cardiol Heart Fail. 2:335–343

Strandberg TE, Sirola J, Pitkälä KH, Tilvis RS, Strandberg AY, Stenholm S (2012) Association of midlife obesity and cardiovascular risk with old age frailty: a 26-year follow-up of initially healthy men. Int J Obes (Lond). 36:1153–1157

Strandberg TE, Pitkälä KH, Tilvis RS, O'Neill D, Erkinjuntti TJ (2013) Geriatric syndromes–vascular disorders? Ann Med 45:265–273

Veronese N, Cereda E, Stubbs B, Solmi M, Luchini C, Manzato E et al (2017) Risk of cardiovascular disease morbidity and mortality in frail and pre-frail older adults: results from a meta-analysis and exploratory meta-regression analysis. Ageing Res Rev 35:63–73

Warwick J, Falaschetti E, Rockwood K et al (2015) No evidence that frailty modifies the positive impact of antihypertensive treatment in very elderly people: an investigation of the impact of frailty upon treatment effect in the HYpertension in the Very Elderly Trial (HYVET) study, a double-blind, placebo-controlled study of antihypertensives in people with hypertension aged 80 and over. BMC Med 13:78

Williamson JD, Supiano MA, Applegate WB et al (2016) Intensive versus standard blood pressure control and cardiovascular disease outcomes in adults aged >75 years. A randomized clinical trial. JAMA 315:2673–2682

Index

N. Veronese (ed.), *Frailty and Cardiovascular Diseases*, Advances in Experimental Medicine and Biology 1216, https://doi.org/10.1007/978-3-030-33330-0

CPSIA information can be obtained
at www.ICGtesting.com
Printed in the USA
LVHW061714120120
643358LV00004B/131/P

9 783030 333294